By Beth Shaw

_____

Beth Shaw's YogaFit®

YogaLean®

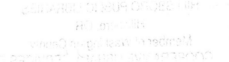

YogaLean®

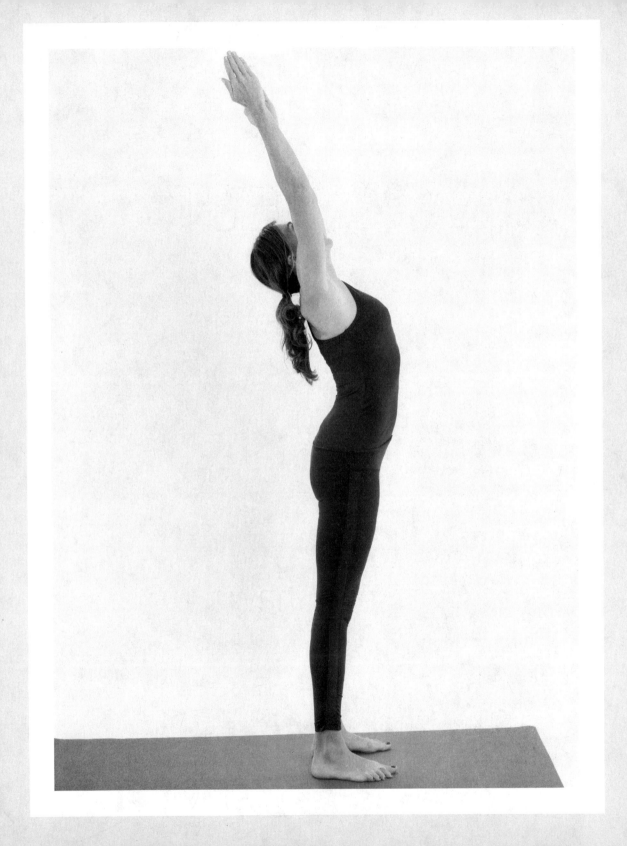

yogalean ®

Poses and Recipes to Promote Weight Loss and Vitality

Beth Shaw

BALLANTINE BOOKS TRADE PAPERBACKS

NEW YORK

A Ballantine Books Trade Paperback Original

Copyright © 2014 by Beth Shaw

Introduction copyright © 2014 by Pam Peeke, M. D.

All rights reserved.

Published in the United States by Ballantine Books,
an imprint of Random House, a division of Random House LLC,
a Penguin Random House Company, New York.

BALLANTINE and the HOUSE colophon are
registered trademarks of Random House LLC.

YOGALEAN is a registered trademark of Beth June Shaw.

YOGAFIT is a registered trademark of Beth June Shaw.

LIBRARY OF CONGRESS CATALOGING-IN-PUBLICATION DATA
Shaw, Beth
Yogalean : poses and recipes to promote weight loss
and vitality—for life! / Beth Shaw.
pages   cm
Includes bibliographical references and index.
ISBN 978-0-8041-7855-6 (paperback) — ISBN 978-0-8041-7856-3 (eBook)
1. Hatha yoga. 2. Reducing exercises. 3. Weight loss.
4. Vitality. 5. Health. I. Title.
RA781.7.S43 2014
613.7'046—dc23   2014024647

5578 6635
9/14

Printed in the United States of America on acid-free paper

www.ballantinebooks.com

2 4 6 8 9 7 5 3 1

Photographs by David Young-Wolff
Book design by Barbara M. Bachman

"Let the beauty you love be the thing that you do."
—*Rumi*

· ·

For the past twenty years I have had the blessing of doing what
I love. From my living room and the trunk of my car in 1994 to offices
in three cities and a presence on six continents, YogaFit® has grown.
This book is dedicated to God, the Universe, a Higher Power,
my Angels, my grandmother Olga, who said that moderation was
the key to everything, my mother, June, who introduced me
to health and fitness at a young age, and my partner, Esra,
for support, courage, and love.

contents

..

foreword

..

fter accepting the invitation to write the foreword to Beth Shaw's *Yoga-Lean*, I spent some time contemplating what it really means to be lean. I discovered that there are many complementary layers to this concept of "lean," each one contributing to the building of a holistic foundation for optimal health and wellness.

Some may hear "lean" and conjure troublesome memories of enduring countless diets in their quest to achieve the Holy Grail of becoming thin. Scale-hopping and obsessing about how to wedge yourself into a size-subzero pair of jeans are clearly not the goals of *YogaLean*. Merriam-Webster defines *lean* as "physically strong and healthy," as in a fit athletic body. To clarify, the goal is not an Olympic career. Rather, *YogaLean* is about each person taking on the project to become as mentally and physically resilient as possible, to survive and thrive joyfully throughout a life of stresses and challenges.

Lean also means to be flexible, inclining from a vertical position, which is the very essence of yoga poses. Physically, you're exploring the extraordinary bounty of flexing, stretching, and strengthening opportunities that yoga gives you. Mentally and spiritually, you're battling the typical dissociation of mind and body that so many experience and that can ultimately lead to self-destructive behaviors, self-abandonment, and a lack of inward awareness. The YogaLean philosophy is a call to action: to cease self-desertion and instead to lean deep into yourself. This is accomplished through the regular and daily practice of this mind-body lifestyle plan, one in which you fearlessly "lean in" and challenge yourself, much like former Facebook CEO Sheryl Sandberg suggests to women seeking career growth in her book of the same name.

Eschewing the traditional diet mentality, *YogaLean* presents a holistic, integrative blueprint based on yogic history and principles. Critical program components are science-based. For example, research now shows that the regular practice of meditation results in astonishing organic changes both in the brain and in how the body's genes direct metabolism. Neuroimaging studies have shown thickening of the brain's cortex in people who meditate regularly, which increases integrative and cognitive thinking. Epigeneticists, who study how genes communicate with one another and commandeer the body's mental and physical functioning, have noted that meditation leads to precise changes in this gene expression, resulting in decreased inflammation and increased mental performance, especially under stressful conditions. Other scientists have discovered that meditation can increase the cell's lifespan, thus increasing longevity. Metabolism specialists have noted a profound and sustained decrease in the stress hormone cortisol following the regular practice of yoga.

Part of honoring the mind and body is to use both. Therefore, physical activity is an integral element in the lifestyle template. Embracing the bliss of movement reinforces the importance of staying connected with the body. This is a serious challenge for stressed-out people, running frenetically 24/7 on the gerbil wheel of overcommitted and overwhelming daily life. It's time to jump off that spinning wheel once and for all and create a new way to live, cherishing and being eternally grateful for each breath we take.

Fueling the daily practice of mindful living with tasty, satisfying, and life-giving whole foods is critical to a healthy lifestyle. New challenges include the need to make the time to shop for, prepare, cook, and gratefully savor each meal. It's a battlefield out there, with endless temptations to skip cooking and instead consume manufactured food-like products that are not natural and pose serious threats to your ability to initiate and maintain healthy behaviors. For example, science has revealed that there is a strong association between certain foods and addiction. Among the chief offenders are processed sugary/fatty/salty food product combinations. Researchers have discovered that, as in drug abuse, we're literally hooked on products like refined sugar. Further, studies published in peer-reviewed journals have demonstrated not only that sugar ignites the brain's reward center in an identical fashion to cocaine, morphine, and heroin but also that, given the option, animals prefer sugary/fatty foods to these drugs. Finally, a milestone study showed that in animals, refined sugar is more addictive than cocaine. Being mindful of every mouthful brings this addictive cycle to a screeching halt.

In focusing on fresh, whole foods while simultaneously encouraging physical movement, the YogaLean program gently transitions people away from the consumption of unnatural products that contribute to disease and physical imbalance and toward an energy-giving appreciation of nutrition that feeds both mind and body wellness.

YogaLean's Four Paths of Yoga are a powerful and accessible way for anyone to understand and appreciate the possibility of his or her own mental, spiritual, and physical transformation. The raja yoga of meditation is, of course, a hallmark of yogic practice. For those of you who think of meditation as foreign or intimidating, think of it as "checking in" with oneself. Everyone is accustomed to checking in with people from their personal and professional sectors in life. When is the last time you checked in with yourself? Many of you, I imagine, would honestly answer "never" or "rarely." How can you understand what your life means, what it will take to change for the better, or how to monitor your daily progress if you don't take the time to go inward regularly?

The second path involves the karma yoga, directing you to pay attention to the importance of service to others. Science shows that when you match your inward journey with an outward reach to help others, your genetic expression changes for the better, decreasing disease risk and promoting optimal health. Jnana yoga, the third path, is a reminder that your personal transformation cannot occur without the knowledge you need to thoroughly understand what must be done. Education provides the key to unlock the door to options and opportunities only new knowledge can give you. Finally, bhakti yoga reinforces the need to devote oneself to the entire practice of mindful self-care. This is an integrative, holistic devotion to your whole self, honoring the miracle of a fully functioning, joyful mind, body, and spirit.

The poet Robert Frost once noted, "The only way out is always through." Yoga-Lean presents a maverick and unique plan to help guide those who know they need to change, are ready to embrace the work, and seek a map to navigate the stormy speed bumps of daily stress. The core goal is to achieve a stronger mind, body, and spirit by confronting and dispelling fears and by shedding the mental weight that impedes personal growth. This "leaner" mind, unburdened by negativity and fueled by empowerment, is open to achieving the physical transformation to a stronger self at the ready to embrace each triumph and challenge with gracious gratitude.

Namaste.

—PAMELA M. PEEKE, MD, MPH, FACP
PEW FOUNDATION SCHOLAR IN NUTRITION
AND METABOLISM
AUTHOR OF THE *New York Times* BESTSELLERS
The Hunger Fix, Body for Life for Women,
AND *Fight Fat After Forty*

introduction

..

"Every block of stone has a statue inside it, and it is the task of the sculptor to discover it."

—MICHELANGELO

Many people assume (as I often do) that when you see someone lean, it is a gift from nature; that they don't struggle with diet or exercise; that their DNA allows for unhealthy choices; and that their naturally blessed metabolism gives them the ability to eat whatever they want, whenever they want. The truth, of course, is that if the "naturally" slender consumed enough fast food, led a sedentary lifestyle, and ignored the instinct that tells each of us to care for our bodies, they would inevitably see (and feel) the effects of their decisions.

I trademarked the name YogaLean in 2002, around the same time I started thinking deeply about the various shapes and sizes of the people around me. How is it that some people are at their "ideal" body weight, while others, despite living similar lifestyles, are not? How does someone's weight spiral completely out of control? Which factors mean the difference between a healthy and an unhealthy lifestyle? In *YogaLean,* the book you're holding in your hands, I address these questions, the general lack of mindfulness in the way we conduct our everyday lives, and how to check yourself before you become overweight or continue to live with unhealthy habits. I provide a program that is easy to implement and easy to follow. YogaLean is a straightforward, no-nonsense plan with proven results, regardless of your current life choices and habits.

Through YogaLean, we learn to gain a sense of our bodies, no matter what our size. We live in "Lean Consciousness," which teaches us how to listen to the needs of our bodies so that we *feel* the difference between optimal health and a life that's unhealthy. Our health is at its best when it is nurtured from a holistic standpoint, practice, belief, and intention.

Like many of you, I have struggled with weight maintenance my entire life. I grew up as a skinny girl who was teased. Due to my height, my classmates called me "ostrich," and I could fit into the jeans of my best friend, who was eight inches shorter.

My parents divorced when I was in eighth grade, and my mother would fill the fridge with cheesecake and pizzas when she left for weekends away. Food became my comfort. By the time I was fifteen, my weight had shot up at least twenty-five pounds. That was when I started going to the gym after school and developed a love for exercise. In college, I met a body builder, who became a good friend. He took me from our upscale health club on Long Island's prestigious North Shore to his grunt-and-sweat gym on the South Shore. There, I met a beautiful female body builder (the first one I'd ever seen), who told me "Don't forget that diet is seventy-five percent of it." This stuck with me forever.

I continued to work out throughout college, but six months later, I left everything in New York behind—including my boyfriend of eight years, my friends, and my family—to move to Los Angeles. Food again became my comfort. I gained forty pounds at a sedentary desk job where I was sleep-deprived, mindlessly typing away on my computer and checking off my "To-Do" list as the workweek slipped away.

Now I am in an industry that requires me to be fit, but it's still not easy! Even though my job is to teach and represent health, fitness, and a lean lifestyle, I have to make a conscious effort every day to balance my schedule with exercise and eating well. If I am not in a state of Lean Consciousness, I quickly put on weight. Therefore, I fill my body and mind every day with good intentions, good food, and good thoughts.

No matter what my schedule looks like—and I am constantly on the road—I always make my body a priority, whether by meditating, working out, hiking, or any other form of movement that gets my heart going. It is my hope that YogaLean will help you fall in love with better choices and movements and spend less time sitting in front of the TV, buying useless items that clutter your life, and engaging in non-productive behavior.

I believe that we all have addictive personalities. The trick to staying healthy is to reprogram your addictions and to choose your habits carefully in order to not cave in.

Here, I provide the tools to gain mental awareness, along with recipes and yoga sequences designed to nurture a leaner body, more energy, stronger immunity, relaxation, and youthfulness. If you follow the YogaLean program, you will transform physically, mentally, emotionally, spiritually, and energetically.

Physically, we will explore tools to help clean up your life and strengthen your body:

Recipes

Yoga poses

Cardio

Weights

Clearing space

Metabolism

Mentally, we will develop a more relaxed mind, one that encompasses positivity and good intentions:

Meditation

New thought patterns

Yamas and niyamas

Essence of yoga

My grandmother Olga Shaw lived to be one hundred and five years old. She cooked her own meals every day, and every evening she took a long after-dinner walk. Her habits were an aid to her longevity. One of my favorite students over the years was Susan, a geriatric nurse at my grandmother's hospital. After getting to know me, Susan approached me with questions about the extra weight she was carrying and her constant fatigue. It had been years since she had exercised, and she wondered what she could do to recover the joy in her life. We started off slowly, by journaling her eating habits, and then we examined them and decided what needed to change. I worked with her on gradually implementing yoga practice, cardio, and meditation in her daily life. Susan lost more than a hundred pounds. If Susan was able to retrain her body to move with intention and grace, so can you.

The YogaLean steps will help rebuild the body temple, regardless of its present state. We will go on a journey from the kitchen to the universe, all the while addressing the body, mind, and psyche to help you stay in sync. YogaLean provides basic yoga poses for better balance, flexibility, and mental and physical strength, and teaches how to clean and organize your kitchen for maximum efficiency and practice meditation to bring you focus and clarity. The ancient yogis said, "Let the stomach be filled with one part food, one part liquid, and one part air." You can access your body's natural state of good health by clearing away the clutter and allowing the light to shine through and outward. With the practice and philosophy of yoga, you will gain a better handle on your body and mind.

When we are balanced in all areas of our life, it becomes easier, if not effortless, to lose and maintain a proper weight. With an understanding that there is an infinite variety of body types, you can let go of judgment, expectation, and competition. You may be inspired to give away or get rid of excess possessions that no longer serve you. You will naturally clear mental space through the practice of meditation and find the freedom to "be."

YogaLean isn't just a practice of health, fitness, balance, and yoga—it is a lifestyle. We become a part of YogaLean, and YogaLean becomes a part of us. The best way to stay YogaLean is to continually practice the techniques and use the tools in this book. You can also download the YogaLean app for iOS or Android to give you additional guidance in putting your learning into practice. It is a great supplement to the book and provides you with additional tools such as healthy recipes, instructions for meditation, helpful day-planning tips, and much more. It is available at the iTunes app store and Google Play.

Don't worry: Anyone can practice YogaLean, and it's okay to start slow or have a lapse in your practice. There's no room for judgment in my studio! It's all about your intentions.

Rather than relying on a strict diet—which, you may know from experience, is often unsustainable over the long term—or avoiding the *why* behind your weight gain, you will move beyond using food as something other than fuel. You'll learn to break the cycle by finding healthier ways to understand your physical and mental needs. Through a combination of current, cutting-edge research and ancient mind/body practices, we will work together to rewire your thinking about how to feed your mind, body, and spirit.

If you stay engaged in the pursuit of YogaLean on a daily basis, you will quickly see results, and the results will be cumulative. It takes twice as much energy to start a car as it does to keep a car running. The same can be said for the YogaLean technique. Getting started will be a challenge, especially if you have neglected your body for years and have let things pile up: weight, addictions, judgments, expectations, possessions. But once you rev that engine, things will start to flow. This is not to say that you will be 100 percent perfect, but you will strive toward maintaining your practice, say, 90 percent of the time. The roadmap of YogaLean will lead you to a beautiful place of balance, peace, and health. You are about to rediscover what you already know deep down: *Nothing* feels better than good health.

Our health is our most valuable asset, always. Stay healthy in a conscious way from this point forward with YogaLean.

Namaste.

PART ONE

. . .

the power
of lean

1

the goal of lean

..

The History of Yoga

Yoga originated in India more than six thousand years ago as a system of psychological and physical practices. These practices create greater health, mental awareness, and balance.

Yoga represents a body of practices that may be fruitfully taken up by anyone who is serious about his or her personal development and aims to build not only a better body but also a life full of greater intention and gratitude as well as a connection to his or her purpose and the universe.

As yoga evolved and expanded, several different variants emerged. In our Western culture, most people are familiar with hatha yoga. Hatha covers all physical yoga, and vinyasa is the fluid style of the movement.

Hatha is a Sanskrit word that means several things. It literally translates to "force" or "physical," but it can be broken down poetically into *ha* and *tha*. *Ha* represents the masculine, solar, or energizing qualities, and *tha* represents the feminine, lunar, or relaxing qualities. The word *hatha* invokes the balance of opposites.

Yoga is the union of opposites through physical practices. Ancient practitioners used the system of hatha yoga as preparation for long periods of sitting. This is why many hatha yoga movements focus on the lower body, especially the hips, hamstrings, and back. Almost all styles of yoga share the same poses. In YogaFit, we use these poses to help create balance in the body and complement the activities of our daily lives.

Physically, yoga massages the skeletal system that supports bone mass and growth while taking the stress away from the supporting muscles and tendons. Yoga mechanically removes tension from the muscles through stretching. Emotionally, the body believes what the mind believes. Affirmations about peace, calm, and tranquility, along with positive imagery, are conveyed to the nervous system. Yoga brings greater relationship with others, life, and ourselves as well as awareness of the emotional blocks that limit our experience of life. Our perception of life has been conditioned by our experiences, and sometimes we close ourselves off from feelings and emotions.

Yoga is tried and true, like a black dress or a white cotton T-shirt, and will never go out of style. It's not a fad diet or workout program; it's an ancient practice aimed at ultimate health and vitality, and it has stuck around for a reason—it works, incorporating philosophy and lifestyle with food, supplements, and, of course, exercise. It is more popular than ever because in this hectic, information-driven, stressful world, it offers a respite through its poses and workouts, which enhance strength, cardiovascular condition, balance, and flexibility, and that in turn creates a sound and stable emotional being and reduces tension and fatigue through mindfulness, fluid movement, and deep breathing focus.

My company, YogaFit, is the largest yoga school in North America, and began as an instructor-training program. When I started teaching yoga in the early 1990s, I found that the traditional methods didn't address the variety of body types, skill levels, and personalities I encountered in my classes. So I developed a user-friendly brand of yoga, YogaFit, that follows the group-exercise model of warmup, work, and cool down. YogaFit offers seminars, educational materials, training manuals, and a series of creative workout videos, yoga apparel, and products.

Every YogaFit instructor is required to complete community service as part of their certification, and students are encouraged to do the same, as giving back helps strengthen your overall happiness as a human being.

YogaFit, using hatha, focuses on linking poses to create strength, flexibility, endurance, and balance—the technique of vinyasa means "to place in a special way." We create classes that effectively work all parts of the body equally, creating an experience of nonjudgment and noncompetition for our students. In *YogaLean*, we'll apply those practices to develop a sense of nonjudgment and noncompetition within ourselves. We aim to take the teachings off the mat and broaden them to create a shift in our real lives, to find that deeper connection within ourselves. The YogaFit Essence, the Four Paths of Yoga, and the foundation of yoga—the yamas and niyamas, which are a set of ten ethical guidelines—help us to develop Lean Consciousness and a well-rounded YogaLean body and mind life. YogaLean is a holistic practice of integrated wellness.

In a society of high-tech, fast-paced overachievers, we all need to reconnect with ourselves: body, mind, and spirit. This healing exercise science brings energy, strength, flexibility, and balance to our physical bodies. Yoga reduces stress and tension in the mind, calming, clearing, and focusing our thoughts. Space is then created for more spiritual awakenings and revelations. As we make rapid gains in technology, people are working longer hours, spending more time in front of computers, and becoming more disconnected from themselves and others as a result.

Yoga can be considered technology for getting back in touch with our true essence and ourselves. It is a way of remembering the health and wholeness that comprise our natural state of being. Yoga, when broken down to its simplest form, is breathing and feeling. Through this breathing and feeling we learn to control our reactions to events and people. It is not the events and people in our lives that give us stress but the way we react to them.

Through yoga we learn to bring awareness to all parts of ourselves with the understanding that through integration, we come to a natural place of balance.

"If you don't know where you are going, you will never get there."

I've included action items throughout this book. One of the most important actions you will make is to write things down, to journal. To achieve a goal, you must first know what your goal is, and you must write down your goals to achieve them. Acknowledging a goal allows you to intentionally move a thought into action in order to improve the quality of your life.

Setting goals down on paper, preferably in a little notebook you carry everywhere, allows you to be free of the thoughts nagging at your conscience. I always keep a notebook with me, and the act of writing things is very powerful, more so than simply typing into your smartphone. When I started YogaFit I wrote down my goals and taped them to the wall where I could see them. Each one came true. Once a goal is written, you can reflect on it on a regular basis, and it becomes easier to manifest. Now you are free from constant thoughts of your goal, and you are then able to *live your goals* naturally.

In *Flow: The Psychology of Optimal Experience*, author Mihaly Csikszentmihalyi describes happiness as being one with your "flow state": a state of concentration so focused that your mind, body, and spirit hone in on a single activity. Many of the activities in this book are best enjoyed in a flow state—exercising, cooking, clearing space, meditating, and, of course, doing yoga. When you write down your goals, you will worry less and enjoy more.

According to Csikszentmihalyi, when you are in a flow state, you feel strong, alert, in effortless control, unself-conscious, and at the peak of your abilities. For instance, if you are in a flow state while pursuing a goal, cooking, exercising, or meditating, you are 100 percent committed to that task, escaping from distractions and negative burdens. Setting and tracking goals is something you can control, strive for, and experience divine pleasure from because it is not left to chance. Instead, goals are purposeful.

"Optimal experience, where we feel a sense of exhilaration, a deep sense of enjoyment that is long cherished, does not come through passive, receptive, relaxing times," he says. "The best moments usually occur when a person's body or mind is stretched to its limits in a voluntary effort to accomplish something difficult and worthwhile."

Everything that manifests in your life is a result of your explicitly acknowledged goals. One common mistake people make is to say that they do not have a vision. *Everyone* has a vision. Use meditation and exercise to tap into it. Yoga and meditation balance the right and left sides of the brain to help you visualize creatively. I often find answers while meditating, practicing yoga, and walking. Tap into that vision and set a goal, one that is real to you and achievable.

What is your goal, and how will YogaLean help you? If it is to lose ten pounds, then you must consciously take steps to achieve that. Start by envisioning yourself at that weight, then write that goal on a Vision Board along with inspirational photos, and place it someplace where you will see it every day. Every time you walk past it, your subconscious mind sees it as a vision. If your vision is strong and your commitment is real, you will take the steps that lead you to it.

Successful people think about the things they want to accomplish. For instance, healthy people think about engaging in activities—proper diet, exercise, and rest—that will bring about health. Visualization is a wonderful power. It can generate warmth or heat, and you can use the power of visualization consciously and continuously to create the kind of future you want for yourself.

Our brains are very complex, and each part has a role in our lives and achieving our goals:

- The left brain is responsible for our conscious awareness and our thoughts.
- The right brain is responsible for our creativity, all sorts of rhythmic behavior, and putting together memory into usable chunks.

- The midbrain is responsible for the energy that powers us in getting things done and in creating memories, while understanding real or imagined emotions.
- The brainstem is responsible for physical stimulus response, for jerking our hand away from a hot stove, for picking up a donut and putting it in our mouth, for lacing up our running shoes.

When these four parts aren't in agreement on an objective, it becomes more difficult to achieve. It's like a football team on which each player is running a different play. Once all four parts of the brain are in agreement, you will have made major progress.

One of the best ways to figure out your goals and track them is through journaling. In YogaLean, you will become very friendly with your journals. Writing in a journal allows you to see, physically, what is going on in your left brain—home of emotions and feelings—as well as the concrete workings of the right brain, such as tracking the food you eat and the goals you hope to achieve. Journaling creates a sense of accountability by making you transcribe your thoughts and actions. I have several notebooks with me at all times—one for feelings and affirmations, one to record my eating habits, and one for my daily, weekly, and life visions and goals.

I separate my journals because I do not want to tangle my right brain with my left. I like to open each journal with a clear intention of what I will be writing. Journaling allows us to tune in to that still, small voice within. As with meditation, there are many ways to use a journal, and I encourage you to try as many as possible to discover which ones are the most effective for you. Below are the journals I hope you implement in your daily routine and use throughout the YogaLean process to put practice to paper.

Daily Notebook: Your Little Catchall Notebook

I carry this with me for daily use: It contains lists, goals, thoughts, quotes, budgets, and to-do lists. You can transfer your notes into your other notebooks if you like.

I prefer a 3" x 5" spiral-bound notebook with a plastic cover so that you can throw it into your laptop case, gym bag, pocket, or purse.

Food Journals

A proven tool that doesn't require another person's involvement is a food journal. "Although compliance can be difficult, ongoing self-monitoring of caloric or fat intake is clearly a correlation of weight-loss maintenance," reports the American Council on Exercise in its "Lifestyle and Weight Management Consultant Manual."

Often we snack at work, or even while preparing a meal, without being aware of how many extra calories we are putting in our body. Keeping a record allows us not only to identify when we are eating mindlessly but also to discover patterns to our eating—whether related to emotional or environmental circumstances.

Personal Journals

Personal journals are an incredibly powerful yet simple means of processing events and circumstances in our lives, healing emotional wounds, and moving forward with passion and intention. Our return to health and well-being often involves being willing to feel in order to heal. The blank page is a safe, objective audience for fielding memories, thoughts, and emotions, rational or irrational. It holds our hand as we dive into exploring the subconscious and does not pass judgment.

Many fields, including yoga, advocate journaling to come to terms with repressed memories, and confusing or traumatic events. Turn off the internal editor, set a timer for ten or fifteen minutes, and write whatever comes to mind. Allow your emotions, thoughts, and energy to flow onto the page, unchecked by judgments or expectations. You'll be amazed what is revealed through the act of "letting go," along with the sense of release that overcomes you.

Other Ways to Journal

Recording inspiration: Write down quotes, poems, advice, and "aha" moments that come your way. This creative act is healing and will give legs to your intentions.

Prayers: Writing down your prayers is an act of surrender, the fifth niyama (see page 27), and ultimate relinquishing of control.

Positive affirmations: Writing your positive affirmations reinforces what yoga calls your *sankalpa,* or positive resolve. It also allows you to go back and reflect on your personal growth and success.

Once you have your journals, you will be able to nail down your goals and engage yourself in the flow state. Stuart Lichtman's "Cybernetic transposition method of goal setting" gives the following steps:

1. Focus on what you consciously want by writing a description. This explicitly frames your conscious intent.

2. While you are thinking about whether you can and will achieve what you want, be alert for any uncomfortable feelings. If and when you experience any, describe them in writing. This explicitly frames any signs of unconscious conflict.

3. Read over your written description of what you want, and identify the specific words or phrases that trigger these signs of unconscious conflict.

4. Underline or circle the words or phrases that cause these feelings. This explicitly frames what triggers the unconscious conflict.

5. Rewrite the words or phrases that you have marked. In this very familiar editing process, you are instructing your unconscious to do what it has often done before: to invent alternatives to what you first recorded.

6. State the words in the present tense. An affirmation is more effective when stated in the present tense. For example: "I now have a wonderful job." Avoid affirming something in the future tense—"I am going to have a wonderful job"—or the results will always be waiting to happen.

"Mastery comes from confidence. Confidence comes from experience. Experience comes from practice. Practice comes from commitment. And commitment comes from vision."

—RANDY GAGE

Mastery is not a place but a process. When you first begin to strive toward a goal, you need to evaluate yourself. What kind of vision do you have for yourself? Be honest. Is it positive, neutral, or negative? Do you have different types of visions for different areas of your life? Look for incongruence here.

One of the best formulas for positive thinking I ever learned was that no matter what is going on around you, think about your goals. Tap into flow state and eventually, through deep concentration and repetition, you will find yourself vividly imaging them. Your subconscious mind can't tell the difference between something that you hope for—a goal, a dream—and a real experience. For example, say your goal is learning to cook. When you envision yourself in the kitchen, twirling around with your apron and stirring a simmering pot of your favorite soup, you're creating the feeling of enjoyment that would accompany you being a master cook. Your subconscious mind simply accepts that you are the best chef in your neighborhood. It doesn't argue with that vision; it doesn't complain; it doesn't try to change your instructions. It simply tries to make your instructions a reality.

Four Dimensions of Visualization

1. *Vividness.* The more vividly you can see something that you want in your mind's eye, the more rapidly it will materialize in your reality. Most people have only a vague, fuzzy picture of what they want. They say they want to be rich or healthy or happy. But when you ask them exactly what that means to them, they don't really know.

> *Your subconscious mind immediately goes to work to coordinate all your resources, internal and external, to bring those desires into your life.*

2. *Intensity.* This refers to the amount of emotion you accompany your mental pictures with. Emotion is central to all accomplishments. There is a little formula: $T \times F = R$, or Thought times Feeling equals Realization. Those people whose lives don't improve from year to year are

those who have never thought about why they want their lives to improve in the first place. If you don't think about the reasons why, you can't generate the emotional excitement and energy that motivate you to do the things that make your dreams come true.

> *One of the most important exercises in visualization is getting the feeling. This means that you imagine something you would like to be, have, or do. Then imagine that you have already accomplished it, and you create the emotion that would accompany the accomplishment of the goal. As you bask in those feelings, like a sunbather basks in the sun, the mental picture is combined with the emotion and passed on to your subconscious mind. Suddenly, amazing things will begin to happen.*

3.   *Frequency.* This refers to how often you play the mental picture of your desired outcome on the screen of your mind. You must convince your subconscious mind that you really want it by repeating the command, that mental picture, over and over, until it is finally accepted as an absolute instruction for your subconscious mind to act on.

4.   *Duration.* This refers to how long you hold the mental image or picture in your mind at one time. The longer you can hold that picture, combined with emotion and vividness, in your mind, the more rapidly it will be accepted by your subconscious mind. That is why you must think about your goals all the time.

Your goals will change and refine over the course of time, so make sure you are flexible and open to change. As you transform, your goals will as well and, as we say at YogaFit, let go of judgment, expectation, and competition.

2

how to develop lean consciousness

..

"You can outeat any exercise program."

YogaLean is about making a choice to improve your health and your body. It is not about absolutes or deprivation. Rather, it's a lifestyle, one that the French have mastered: They eat real food that's clean and good for you, not highly processed junk. They also walk a lot. As a rule, they don't eat pizza at home in front of the TV or order drive-through and eat in their cars.

I have been inspired by a lot of other lean influencers along the way. One was a competitive cyclist with an amazingly cut body who lived in San Francisco. He used cycling as his primary mode of transportation, working hard to trek up and down the steep hills. At every meal, he ate half his food and preserved the other half, either saving it for dinner or giving it to a homeless person. He practiced this method of portion control to ensure that he did not overeat.

Another lasting influence is a good friend who is a celebrity stylist. As soon as her food is served, she takes half her order and places it in a to-go box for her next meal. Many American restaurants serve enormous portions, so I remember these inspirations every day and split my meal with a friend or remember to ask for a doggy bag before I begin to eat. Portion control is a conscious decision not to over-eat, and guess what? It works.

Developing Lean Consciousness is closely connected with yoga practice. Through the practice of yoga, we develop greater body awareness, which allows us to look at a food item and intuitively know how it will make us feel. That cupcake may look and taste great, but in twenty minutes you will experience a sugar rush, a headache, and fatigue. That second martini may be appealing in the moment, but tomorrow you will feel dehydrated and sluggish. You will learn from experience and make better choices.

We, as humans, are given the opportunity every day. You have the choice to eat breakfast or skip it, to drink that second cup of coffee, or to indulge in an impulse fast-food item. We are never going to be 100 percent perfect, as that would be both boring and compulsive, but 80 to 90 percent of the time, we can choose foods that are fresh and nonprocessed and will make us feel amazing. You must remember that you are lucky and *get to* choose, unlike so many others. If you are reading this book, you have made at least one positive, proactive decision today!

What Is Lean Consciousness, and How Can You Develop It?

Lean Consciousness is a mind/body way of being in which all the decisions and choices you make move you to a state of greater health. Oftentimes the body and the mind are at odds with each other. The mind wants something that is not necessarily good for the body. Our bodies do not naturally crave processed food unless we have had enough of it to get us addicted—and, unfortunately, many of us got hooked young.

In the movie *Super Size Me,* Morgan Spurlock showed us how thirty days of fast food created an altered and addictive state of desire and depravity around food choices.

Addiction is caused when we suppress our feelings. We need to learn how to feel our emotions, rather than hiding or fearing them. Oftentimes the body and mind are looking for breath and energy to feel better, but instead we fill them with food, especially in times of stress. Stress eating helps to soothe us and to make us forget about what is making us feel frazzled, especially comfort foods like pizza and ice cream. If we recognize how to feel rather than feed, it can eliminate our addictions.

Sugar addiction runs rampant in our society but can be cured by eliminating sugar from our diets. This may not stop the cravings altogether, but if you can use yoga and meditation to curb them, your body's innate desire to be in a state of optimal health will emerge.

Lean Consciousness enables the body and mind to work together to achieve health goals. Once in a state of Lean Consciousness, you will approach life in a whole new way. Food choices become based on body need—not want. You will begin to eat for energy, immunity, and health, not pleasure, stress, or boredom.

I will teach you how to access Lean Consciousness through meditation and yoga, which calm, center, and focus the mind. Meditation gives us coping skills and creates better functioning of our prefrontal cortex, the executive functioning center of the brain. This leads to healthier choices and less reactivity or eating out of boredom, fear, anger, and restlessness!

Seven Steps to YogaLean

Developing Lean Consciousness takes commitment and perseverance. By transforming our current way of thinking and living to embody healthy choices, we become lean. Change your thoughts, change your mind, change your body.

Aside from the food you eat, your mind also needs to digest purer thoughts for your body to believe that you will succeed. Whether you want to lose weight or stay fit, it is crucial to learn what is good for you and then live by it. Below are my steps to becoming YogaLean and developing a Lean Consciousness.

1. Believe you can transform your body

With hope, trust, and belief, we can achieve our goals, no matter what they are. If you have a deep belief combined with an action plan, you will manifest your goals.

Regardless of your body type, it is important to know in your heart you are not trapped. It may take time, but if you truly want a better, healthier body, you can and *absolutely* will get it. Replacing negative energy with a focus on positive thinking is the first step. Once you believe in yourself, the universe will follow suit.

In *The Alchemist,* Paulo Coelho writes, "When you want something, all the universe conspires in helping you to achieve it." You know why? Because once we acknowledge our desire, we use the tools around us to build the foundation, to make choices that build toward that goal, and to surround ourselves with people who motivate us.

ACTION ITEM

Journal every morning about what you have accomplished in the past day, week, and month.

2. Clear the clutter

What is really getting in the way of your weight loss? Everything in the universe has energy. Sometimes having too much stuff in our lives blocks our energy and creates barriers to success. It's time to filter out the negative energy coming at you, whether it's from people, television, or the news. It is easier to make decisions in a state of calm than in a storm. By literally removing the clutter from our lives, we can remove the clutter from our bodies. Often too many possessions and a "hoarding" mindset leave us with too many unwanted pounds. Try living in a zen space.

Write a list of two things you will do every day
to create space and clear clutter—check your list
every morning when you journal.

3. Create your multifaceted and holistic plan

Visualize the wheel of a bicycle; as you're looking at it, notice that it has many spokes. If one of the spokes is broken, bent, or malfunctioning, the wheel is compromised and can collapse. The YogaLean program is the same way. It involves nutrition, exercise, yoga, meditation, supplementation, positive affirmations, and an action plan that work together for a smooth ride. Your wheel also involves support groups, journaling, and community service work.

Crafting a plan that works for you is crucial, because if you feel bogged down by a plan that doesn't conform to your personality or even your schedule, it will feel and seem (and maybe even *be*) forced and impossible. YogaLean and Lean Consciousness truly enable you to develop a lifestyle that is easy to follow, a plan that allows you to enjoy life to its fullest while maintaining a healthier way of being.

Make a vision board and hang it above your desk or in
your bathroom. Your vision board should include
things you want to accomplish and how you see your
space looking and feeling. If you see this vision board
every day, you will be reminded of what you want.

4. Get comfortable being uncomfortable— learn to love movement

Let's face it—dieting is uncomfortable, and exercise, even yoga, can be as well. In fact, in yoga we put ourselves in very uncomfortable positions in order to learn how to stay present for life's challenges. As Eckhart Tolle says, when faced with a difficult situation you can leave it, accept it, or transform it. Sometimes in life, leaving is just not an option, so we must learn to accept and transform the situation. We cannot leave our bodies.

Many people live in so much fear, rigidity, and resistance that being open is not an option. Even if they are uncomfortable with their weight or a difficult life experience, creating change is scarier. We humans do not like change. But the reality is that everything is always changing, so it's better to get into the river and go with the current than try to hold back the tide with your little paddle. Sometimes you need surrender.

At first, this shift of consciousness might feel foreign, scary, and uncomfortable, but once your body adapts, it will feel like the norm. If we live a life trying to avoid challenges, we will become stagnant, piling on things that are weighing us down and not allowing us to evolve or grow (although our pants size might). Life without change is boring. Embrace the idea of a leaner, clearer, and different you!

ACTION ITEM

Do one thing every week or month that makes you uncomfortable—learning a new sport, taking up a hobby, experimenting with a more productive way of doing things, trying a new vegetable or fruit, learning to cook! Write it in your journal as an accomplishment.

5. Be committed and open to doing whatever it takes

Flexibility and commitment are key. If something does not work, you go to plan B. Just because something works one day, that doesn't mean it will work the next. Close your eyes. Remember a time that you really wanted something—a promotion at work, a trip to Europe, a new pair of shoes—and were willing to do whatever it took to get it. Be this way with your health.

You have taken the first step to a healthy life, and that is enormously admirable. Ask yourself where you want your body to be in six months, and do your best to get it there. Keep asking. Your answer will never be, "I want a body that is sluggish."

ACTION ITEM

Meditate on being the person you are inside—
the person that is the best of you, not anyone else.

6. Get a support system

There are going to be people around you who support and people who sabotage. Learn to differentiate between supporters and saboteurs. Support groups can come in many forms: a workout buddy, Overeaters Anonymous groups, yoga friends.

When we start to get healthy, we see things differently. We may notice a friend who drinks too much or is always negative, just as we may learn to appreciate a friend who wants to meet for a hike instead of cocktails. Try this for a month: Instead of meeting your friends for drinks or dinner, schedule them for a hike, a walk, or yoga.

Surround yourself with people who want the same things you do—a healthy body and mind. Nothing is better than a pat on the back or congratulations for your hard efforts. A true friend will do this for you! Also, if your support system knows that you are on this journey, it will help you get out of a rut if you fall into one; it will hold you accountable if you begin to lose sight of your goal; and it will encourage you to stay committed and will hold you high when you reach the finish line.

You are not in this alone. There are people out there who are proud of your change—keep them close!

Talk daily to those who support you—friends,
family, and your team. Make time for a ten-minute call
(or longer) to one support member a day.

7. Forgive yourself

We are human. We make mistakes, we fall down, we get up, and oftentimes, we fall down again. Life is not a linear path; it is more like the roads in India. The first time I went to India, I was amazed at the road from Delhi to Rishikesh, where we hold YogaFit retreats. It's filled with cows, trucks that often break down, rickshaws, motorcycles carrying four people, and bicycles. Sometimes it can take up to ten hours to complete a journey that a glance at a map would indicate should only take four.

This is just like life—bumpy, messy, filled with obstacles. If we fall out of line with our goals, if we devour an entire pizza because we had a bad day, we must forgive ourselves and acknowledge that it was a misstep. The overall good work you are doing toward your goals is what's important. If you do slip up, know that it is not the end of the road but simply a detour.

You are on the path to better health, so work extra hard tomorrow to laugh off mistakes and drive forward with grace, focus, and forgiveness.

ACTION ITEM

Practice a forgiveness meditation for yourself
and others. Allow yourself to honor what happened
and then move on.

The Essence of YogaFit

In our YogaFit trainings, we equip our future instructors with seven steps to help them relate to each student and understand his or her individual challenges. These seven components enable each of us to let go of those things that bog us down mentally and hinder us from moving forward. Incorporating these items into your YogaLean lifestyle will enhance your efforts to develop a cleaner, healthier life.

1. Breathing

The breath is our most powerful tool to relax our bodies and clear our minds. Breathing also allows you to regroup and stay present. Let's say you're having a moment and your brain automatically veers toward what will make you feel comforted: candy, a milkshake, or pastrami on rye with a vat of pickles. Taking a minute to gather yourself with deep breaths will refocus your entire being, allowing you to evaluate what just happened and to refocus on your goals.

Life is fast-paced, and if we give ourselves the space to close our eyes and inhale deeply, filling our body with good thoughts and intentions while slowly exhaling the negative, we will stay on track.

ACTION ITEM

Practice a breathing technique listed in
this book every day.

2. Feeling

We want to feel something in every pose, action, and thought. In yoga, we are always reminded to check in with our bodies in order to modify poses to provide less or more sensation. When we feel something in our bodies, we stay grounded in the moment and in awareness of our body and its potential. The more we learn to feel what's really going on, the less we will make unhealthy choices.

Addiction is a result of avoiding our true emotions. Instead of confronting our feelings, we fill the void with our addiction. Food is perhaps the most widely accepted addiction in our country. Whether it's drugs, alcohol, love, or food, an addict consumes because he or she is disconnected from his or her feelings.

Feeling involves learning to feel full on less food. It also will allow you to understand how bad choices are affecting your life. When you feel bad emotionally and shovel a pint of ice cream into your mouth, then you feel bad physically. Learning to accept and work with your feelings will give you a better sense of how to shift those feelings from negative to positive. Instead of running to the ice cream aisle, we will run to the track to let our body shake off the stress or sadness. Choosing exercise rather than overeating will innately and scientifically make you feel better physically and emotionally. Have you ever regretted exercise? The "runner's high" is real. When we exercise, our body produces endorphins that make us feel lighter, even enlightened. Embrace that feeling. Addiction is caused by suppression of feelings. We need to learn how to feel our emotions rather than fear them; often the body is looking for breath and energy to calm itself, but instead we fill it with food.

ACTION ITEM

Every day, lie down in Final Relaxation pose and
feel all parts of the body.

3. Listening to the Body

Our body tells us everything we need to know. The trick is learning to listen. It knows exactly the foods we need to eat. If you're sick, your body needs a boost of vitamins; that's why we eat soup full of vegetables and healing nutrients. During menstruation, a woman's body fatigues because of the loss of iron, so she may crave meat. When we need energy, our body wants carbs.

As mentioned earlier, we do not naturally desire unhealthy processed foods. Those are cravings of the mind, influenced by TV commercials for pizza, burgers, and products full of white flour and sugar. We need to learn how to differentiate between mental and physical desires in order to evoke a sense of wellness.

Yoga helps us tap into our body's voice and listen to it through meditation and breathing. YogaLean is all about listening to the body and developing a consciousness (a lean one).

ACTION ITEM

Practice turning inward for at least five minutes twice a day. Feel how your body reacted to your day and your meals, and recognize what needs to be done to make it feel better, to feel optimal.

4. Letting Go of Competition

Our bodies are like snowflakes; every one is unique, based on genetics and life experiences. In YogaFit, we do not expect one person to look exactly like another in a yoga pose. As you will see in the next chapter, there are different body types—kapha, vata, and pitta. A kapha person may be mesomorphic and will never be a size 2, whereas a vata person may be endomorphic and naturally lean.

It's time to let go of competition to be the best possible person that you can be—not for anyone else, but for *you*. Compete only against yourself to be your own personal best. This isn't about winning, it's about achieving.

ACTION ITEM

Instead of wanting to be or beat others, make a plan to be your best you—write down five of your strongest qualities or five accomplishments you achieved that day. It can be anything from "I drank eight glasses of water today" to "I got a promotion." Focus on every positive thing you did that day.

5. Letting Go of Judgment

It's important to let go of judgment if you have a challenging day and fail to meet a goal. Judging yourself and others stops individuality and self-growth. It's easy to judge yourself if you are trying to hold to a strict diet. Forgiveness is paramount. If you fall off your eating program one day, just move on and get back on it tomorrow.

We are human and not perfect. Allow acceptance to replace judgment, and learn from the mistake rather than judging it.

ACTION ITEM

Make amends. Notice when you judge another—
write it down and commit to altering that behavior.
When you judge, catch it and send an apology to
that person out loud to the universe—he or she does
not have to hear it. You can also write it down and
then throw it away. This will allow you
to recognize what you did and thought.

6. Letting Go of Expectations

As I always say, "It's called yoga *practice* for a reason—not yoga perfection."

In yoga, we turn our attention inward. Encouraging ourselves to let go of external comparisons and judgments allows us to have a deeper experience in our practice. Learn to let go of your expectations; practice based on how you feel *today,* not how you felt in your last yoga class. Yoga is a process and a journey, not a destination.

Naturally, if you have high expectations and those expectations are not met, you will feel down and disappointed. I don't want you ever to feel disappointed in yourself if you are trying your best, so try to let go of any impossible standards you're carrying around and live in the present moment.

Did something not go your way?
Did you fail yourself?
Reframe it so that you realize you are doing
the best you can for you.

7. Staying in the Present Moment

Living in the now means in this moment everything is okay. It means that whatever happened yesterday is behind us and gone. Don't beat yourself up for the choices you made during lunch. Whatever happens tomorrow is not here, nor is it guaranteed. When practicing YogaLean, try to make healthy choices in each moment—with the understanding that healthy moments are cumulative and will add up to a healthy person, just like a lifetime of unhealthy moments lead to a sick person. You *can* start making healthy choices in this very moment.

There is a study called "Popcorn Amnesia" that shows that when people eat, their minds focus on the act of chewing. Our brain tells our mouth and its muscles to chew, and that takes up valuable mental real estate. If you are eating while reading or working at your desk, your body is consuming calories rather than information. Take the time to slow down and separate your actions, focusing on the task at hand. One of the most damaging and most common things I see is people scrolling through their phone while interacting with another human being. It's time to live one moment at a time. Appreciate what you're putting into your body. Focus on doing the best work you possibly can. And put your phone down when people are talking to you.

Notice how many times a day you go to the past
or the future. Catch yourself—write it down and do a
present-moment-awareness breathing technique.
Create and use the mantra "Be here now."
Ask yourself: What is my intention for today?
How will I be healthier? How can I better
observe my feelings today?

The Eight Limbs of YogaLean

In yoga, the goal is to become a cleaner person, both physically and mentally, in order to serve the world and our life with great purpose and meaning. There are tools and techniques, aside from the physical act of going to class, that guide us toward health and intentionality.

The traditional limbs to help us better understand how yogis observe life and themselves:

1 and 2. **YAMAS AND NIYAMAS** serve as a Ten Commandments of sorts for moral and ethical conduct and self-discipline.

- **YAMAS refer to the physical acts or the five abstentions, how we relate to the external world:**

  a) Ahiṃsā: nonviolence and inflicting no injury or harm to others and one's own self. It also asks that we refrain from violence in thought, word, and deed.

   b) **Satya:** truth; non-illusion and remaining true in our words and thoughts.

   c) **Asteya:** not coveting things in the possession of others and ourselves; not stealing.

   d) **Brahmacharya:** moderation in all things, and using our energy to move forward in our goal of reaching the truth, suggesting that our relationships should foster our understanding of the highest truths.

   e) **Aparigraha:** non-possessiveness; non-hoarding.

- **NIYAMAS refer to the five observances, how we relate to ourselves and the inner world**

   f) **Shaucha:** cleanliness of body and mind.

   g) **Santosha:** satisfaction with what one already has; contentment.

   h) **Tapas:** austerity and associated observances for body discipline and thereby mental control.

   i) **Svādhyāya:** study of the Vedic scriptures on God and the soul, which leads to introspection on a greater awakening to the soul and God within.

   j) **Īśvara-Praṇidhāna:** surrender to (or worship of) God.

3. **ASANA:** self-discipline of the body through the yoga poses; using them correctly and intentionally to aid in our health.

4. **PRĀṆĀYĀMA:** control of life force energies through breathing, recognizing the connection between intentional breathing and the mind and emotions.

5. **PRATYAHARA:** the ability to step back and take a look at ourselves, allowing us to observe objectively the cravings and habits that are detrimental to our health and inner growth.

6. **DHĀRAṆĀ:** concentration on a single object, such as a star in the sky, in order to hone in on our ability to tame the mind and control it; this limb naturally assists with our growth in meditation (below).

7. **DHYĀNA**: meditation.
8. **SAMĀDHI**: physical connection, or oneness, with the results of meditation. Transcending beyond thought and concentration and becoming tied with the universe through bliss and a state of ecstasy.

The Eight Limbs of YogaLean are a holistic approach to weight loss, combining ancient wisdom with current research on the science of weight loss and behavior modification with the goal of achieving wellness of the mind, the body, and the spirit. They offer the greatest opportunity for total transformation, allowing you to be fully present to your life's purpose and potential—from understanding what holds this practice together to how to apply it in our daily lives.

YogaLean Limb 1: Yamas and Niyamas

"Practice with the body you have today."

Just as the "essence of YogaFit" is the heart of YogaFit teachings; the yamas and niyamas are the soul. Think of these as a map to get from one destination to the next. These ten principles can lead you to a healthier life, which includes journaling and practicing asanas (poses), inspire the manifestation of thoughts via positive affirmations, and motivate you toward mindfulness. Once growth begins, it never stops. It may slow or even stall for a time, but if you choose to apply these principles to your life today, they will transform you tomorrow and throughout your life.

YAMAS

Yamas are the physical principles that involve ways of speaking, eating, and breathing to lead to a YogaLean body.

- **AHIMSĀ**: the practice of nonviolence toward yourself and other living beings.

  This applies to our thoughts and actions in the way we treat our body, avoiding violence. We should refrain from eating disorders or starving ourselves and from overtaxing our body with alcohol, fried fatty foods, excess sugar, or other unhealthy substances. Traditional yogis choose a vegetarian diet because the consumption of meat is violence toward animals. Every recipe in this book is vegetarian, but there are suggested add-ins for those of you who opt for animal proteins.

- **SATYA**: the practice of truthfulness.

  Satya is honesty in speech, thoughts, and deeds with the consistent intention to heal or help, not hurt. In order to achieve any goal, there are two major factors, to begin with: where we are and where we want to be. There can be some flexibility in determining where we want to be, but identifying where we are currently requires brutal, rigid honesty that can only come from ourselves.

  Being honest with yourself and with others will give you a truthful foundation to work from. If something is wrong and you recognize it honestly, you can fix it. If you have a weakness, make it into a strength. If you are eating poorly, be honest about the harm you are causing.

  Food journaling will help you hold yourself accountable for your actions. Write down what you're eating or addicted to and see what needs to change.

- **ASTEYA**: the practice of taking only what belongs to us—discerning and seeking only what we need versus what we want.

  It takes time to understand the difference, but you can begin practicing asteya by releasing cravings as perceived needs and cultivating a sense of self-sufficiency. You'll begin to reduce food waste or refrain from going to the pantry and eating mounds of food; if you're a parent, you will stop eating the leftovers on your child's plate.

  In YogaFit we say, "Listen to your body." That gut feeling, the one that physically hurts when something is wrong, is telling you something. When you are stressed, your body may ache. When you eat a slice of cake, your body may fatigue. Feed yourself with emotions and foods that give your body what it *needs*.

- **BRAHMACHARYA**: the practice of moderation in all areas of life, from food consumption and exercise to sleep and work.

  Remember my bicyclist friend who divides up his food when he eats? That action is a form of moderation. This may feel unattainable at this point in time, but if you apply all the other yamas and niyamas, as well as the rest of the practices that make up YogaLean, moderation will become the rule rather than the exception. As your mind, body, and spirit become healthier, you will begin to draw away from extremes and find comfort in the middle ground.

  Treat your body to a break and give yourself adequate rest from work. Europeans are admirable in that sense, as they "work to live" rather than "live to work." They don't make work their sole purpose in life; rather, they make it their means to a prosperous life, earning money to vacation during the summer. (The Italian government actually provides monetary supplements for vacation. Can you imagine?)

- **APARIGRAHA**: the practice of letting go of all worldly, extraneous items and relationships that we rely on for peace and happiness.

  While there is nothing wrong with possessions and people in our lives, when we *need* them to feel centered and complete, we call them "attachments." For instance, if we are slaves to our cell phones, instead of thinking, we might Google for information. As a culture, we are adopting a device addiction, whereas we got through life just fine without the devices before. I'm not saying to throw your phone away, but try leaving it home when going to dinner with friends and becoming enthralled in the present conversation. Or explore a new city without it, looking up at your new surroundings rather than down at your friend Jill's Facebook status.

  This practice also applies to letting go of those relationships that aren't supporting us and our healthy needs—like the drinking buddy or the fast-food addict.

NIYAMAS

The niyamas are guidelines for how we interact with our internal world. The practice of the niyamas harnesses the energy created through the practice and application of the yamas. While these principles are about our inner life, their impact will reach far beyond us.

- **SAUCHA**: the practice of external and internal purity (cleanliness).

  Your body is a temple and needs to be treated as such. What we put into it affects not just our weight but also our entire endocrine system, which controls energy, mood, mental activity, and stress management. Eating whole organic foods, drinking filtered water, eliminating processed foods and stimulants, and exercising will clear the toxins from our body and our mind.

  Also, if you create a clear and organized space at work and home, including your kitchen, you will be able to focus on living intentionally. When your internal and external environments are treated as sacred space, you invite the sacred into your life.

- **SANTOSHA**: the practice of contentment.

  This principle teaches us how to recognize when we feel full and be content with less. America loves huge portion sizes, and we have adjusted to eating past the point of contentment. Again, the yoga body is one part food, one part air, one part liquid—fill it respectfully and correctly. Learn to be content with less.

- **TAPAS**: the practice of discipline.

  Losing weight isn't about willpower, but it is about staying the course no matter how difficult it may become, whether that means waking up early to exercise, doing ten more pushups even when your arms are on fire, feeling emotional discomfort instead of reaching mindlessly for a snack (or your phone to distract yourself), or connecting with a truth you have been denying.

  Tapas literally means "heat" or "fire," which refers to our internal fire—our digestion. Fuel the fire and your metabolism by eating spicy foods and other nutrients and minerals; this promotes a healthy "fire." Practicing tapas also includes a continual exercise regimen. Consider engaging tapas before going back for that second plate of food.

- **SVĀDHYĀYA**: the practice of self-observation.

  This is the path of self-education and study through internal awareness and external resources. By learning to step back and breathe, you will better understand your own reactions and what triggers them, which will help you become conscious of how you are treating yourselves. Again, instead of running for the ice cream to soothe your stress, run the path of nature, letting your shoes on the ground stomp the feeling.

Take an honest inventory of yourself and your weaknesses. Even the best driver has a blind spot. Find that blind spot and commit to understanding it. If you have a problem with your weight, what do you need to do to solve that problem?

By cultivating a spirit of exploration, we open ourselves to answers from within as well as through books, teachers, and circumstances that seem to appear at just the right moment. Remember, the universe is on our side and will present things to us when we need them in order to help us on our journey.

- **ĪŚVARA-PRAṆIDHĀNA: the practice of surrender.**

This principle centers not on us but on God, divinity, and the light that shines *within* all of us. Through the practices of YogaLean, we will slowly begin to unclench our physical, mental, and spiritual restraints in order to receive our birthright of peace, joy, and health. Surrender what is out of your control, and begin to do the work set before you with faith, trust, hope, and love.

Find whatever it is that helps you feel connected, whether it's nature, art, music, literature, yoga, meditation, or anything else that calms your soul.

By practicing YogaLean, you are surrendering your weight loss to a higher power and using Lean Consciousness to guide you on your path to health and happiness.

ACTION ITEM

In a journal, write down your strongest connection
to one yama and niyama. Write down also where
you need to increase strength.

YogaLean Limb 2: Meditation

"Flirt with meditation until you marry it."

There's an old Zen saying: "You should sit in meditation for twenty minutes a day, unless you're too busy; then you should sit for an hour."

Meditation affords us an opportunity to take a step back, breathe, and evaluate our inner soul. It's easy to put all your energy into losing weight to the point where it becomes a burden rather than a goal. Meditation lets us relax, and evaluate ourselves and our progress; the benefits to our physical, emotional, mental, and spiritual well-being are astounding. It promotes internal awareness and acceptance—an opportunity to observe objectively instead of reacting to daily events, both positive and negative—and allows us to recognize the totality of our responses to potentially toxic emotions, such as anger, guilt, fear, and grief.

YogaLean will help you implement meditation practice every day.

ACTION ITEM

Practice at least ten minutes daily—if pressed for time,
do this when you wake up or before you go to sleep.

YogaLean Limb 3: Breathing

"Breath is spirit, so let's breathe big."

Because we breathe every moment of our lives, it's easy to take it for granted. But when we do take the time to tap into the pattern of our breathing, it has a profound effect. Our breath affects our nervous system and is connected to our stress response. For example, when our breathing is short and shallow, it increases stress hormones, including cortisol and adrenaline, which can lead to spikes in blood sugar and increased weight gain, particularly in the abdominal region. Try it right now—how does that feel? Like you're nervous, right? Anxious?

Now try this—long inhale and deep exhale. Instantly, this invokes a relaxation response in the body.

Breathing is the key to mindfulness, emotional clarity, and physical awareness.

Becoming one with our breath enhances energy, increases metabolism, and allows us to feel, heal, and be present to this moment.

Practice one breathing technique daily for at least five minutes.

YogaLean Limb 4: Positive Affirmations

"Let's err on the side of the light."

Our thoughts provide the soundtrack for our lives. According to the National Science Foundation, the average person has about twelve thousand thoughts a day. The thoughts that travel in our mind shape us and give us the beat to walk to. You are what you think.

Ponder this for a second: How many of your thoughts are negative criticisms you hear from others? Or judgments you pass and dwell on? How are these influencing you? These heavy thoughts will give you heavy boots and become a part of your personal soundtrack.

Affirmations need to be stated in the most positive terms possible. Avoid negative statements. Affirm what you do want, rather than what you don't want. For example: "I am no longer unhealthy" is a negative statement. Instead, affirm that "I am now perfectly healthy in body, mind, and spirit." This statement is much more powerful, as it is positive, reinforces your desired goal, and doesn't confuse your subconscious mind with the mention of the undesirable condition.

The mechanics that make affirmations powerful are:

- REPETITION: Repeating imprints the affirmation into your subconscious mind.
- EMOTIONS: Get involved, be passionate, and use your emotions. Think carefully

about the meaning of the words as you repeat them rather than just writing, typing, or saying them.

- **PERSISTENCE**: Practicing affirmations with persistence achieves results much sooner than practicing them periodically. Successive sessions will have a compounding effect.
- **BELIEF**: You need the ability to *feel* what it would be like when the desire you're affirming is fulfilled. Every time that you have a need—and that need is met—a certain "feeling" is produced in you.
- **IMPRESS YOURSELF**: Personalize your affirmations. They must *resonate* with you—feel right for you. The stronger your connection with the affirmation, the deeper impression it makes on your mind, and the sooner you will experience positive results.

Through meditation and the practices taught here, you have the opportunity to rewrite your negative thinking and focus on the positive things that are constantly blossoming around you. Every day, compliment yourself, and while you're at it, compliment someone else.

ACTION ITEM

Write positive affirmations on Post-it notes and put them on your makeup or bathroom mirror— say them out loud so that you are physically connected to your positive thoughts.

YogaLean Limb 5: Exercise

"The body wants to move, the mind may or may not."

Exercise, particularly yoga practice, helps us to develop a healthy relationship with our body. In *A Course in Weight Loss,* Marianne Williamson calls exercise "an aspect of the right relationship with your body, something you give to it in exchange for all it does for you. Your body *wants* to move; movement helps your muscles, your heart, your lungs, and your brain. Give your body what it really wants, and it will give to you what *you* really want."

Yoga includes attention to the breath, mindfulness, gratitude, and growing the positive mind, which all benefit long-term weight management. If you treat your body well, it will feel better, and your mind will follow suit with an improvement to self-esteem and body image.

It's important to also practice tapas and self-discipline. Movement is important for stimulating circulation through the lymphatic system, which is a central component of our body's trash collection and purification systems. Build up a sweat; it helps stimulate detoxification.

EXERCISE AND YOUR ENDOCRINE SYSTEM

Our hormones are largely responsible for weight gain, but exercise is a powerful antidote because it regulates hormones that are out of check. An energetic workout will reduce cortisol (a stress hormone that causes weight gain and other health issues), release fat-burning growth hormone, make cells more sensitive to insulin (which decreases blood sugar and prevents weight gain), and even increase metabolism-boosting thyroid hormones. Exercise stimulates production of the hormone DHEA along with your endorphins, which teams up with your adrenal glands to give you more energy, increase your libido, and help alleviate depression. It's that "runner's high" again.

Yoga, when compared to other forms of exercise, such as cardio, preferentially increases levels of the neurotransmitter GABA (gamma-amino butyric acid), which regulates the activity of the nerves. People with anxiety, depression, or other mood disorders often have lower levels of GABA, and yoga practice has been demonstrated to increase those levels in the thalamus, which benefits our feelings of well-being and reduces anxiety. Ultimately, a stable mind allows the spokes on our wheel to function together, giving us the opportunity to make better food choices.

How Much Is Enough?

Exercise or movement of some sort should be incorporated into most days of the week, if not every day, depending on the intensity of your workouts. While some weight loss theories advocate high-intensity workouts, I believe that regular moderate-intensity yoga practice, cardio, and weight training, combined with the other YogaLean principles, are sufficient to promote healthy weight loss (1 to 2 pounds a week) and boost energy, mood, and self-efficacy—all critical to achieving and maintaining a healthy weight.

ACTION ITEM

Make a plan to do some sort of exercise daily. I advocate seven 30- to 90-minute sessions a week of yoga, cardio, weights, hiking, walking, or an additional hobby sport. The trick is to learn to love to move.

YogaLean Limb 6: Support

*"Surround yourself only with people who
support your highest good."*

As I mentioned in the "Seven Steps to YogaLean," a support system is undeniably crucial. Our brains contain neurons that reflect the emotions of the people surrounding us, and it is imperative as we set an intention to change our lives that we spend time with "healthy" people who inspire and support our efforts. One of the predominant predictors of success in losing weight and keeping it off is support from the key players in your life. Don't be afraid to ask for it, and don't be afraid to seek it out. Your family and good friends are there to cheer you on in your life journey.

Daniel Amen, author of *Change Your Brain, Change Your Body,* cites a study published in *The New England Journal of Medicine* that shows one of the strongest associations in the spread of obesity is who you spend time with. If you have a friend who is obese, you have a 57 percent higher chance of becoming obese yourself—and a 171 percent higher chance if that person is considered a close friend. "It is not a new virus that has been discovered," he writes, "but the social and behavioral influence of your friends."

Imagine you have a friend who eats burgers every day and one who eats salads. If you hang around the burger fiend, you are more susceptible to eating burgers. If you spend your time with the salad advocate, you will naturally also eat salads. You really want someone who will understand your goals and help you achieve them without putting them to any trouble.

ACTION ITEM

Connect with a member of your "support team" daily,
whether it be via text or phone call.

YogaLean Limb 7: Journaling

"We learn who we are by observing our behaviors."

In addition to support, accountability and record keeping are paramount when it comes to healthy weight loss.

ACTION ITEM

Many of the action items and takeaways in this book
require journaling—buy three journals, one for food,
one for personal thoughts, and one for everything
else. Make sure you are writing everything down.

YogaLean Limb 8: Nutrition

Most of us with weight issues have lost touch with how to nurture our bodies and souls with food. Our relationship with food has become complex and often dysfunctional. Rather than eating for fuel or enjoying the experience of a meal with family and friends, we've turned to food to soothe us when we feel hurt, comfort us when we are in need of solace, celebrate joy, or protect us when we feel vulnerable. We may even use food to help us feel grounded if we've been "in our heads" too much, if we're sedentary, or if we're spending hours commuting or sitting at a desk.

Or, for chronic dieters, we've come to depend on depriving ourselves in order to "achieve" health and the "perfect" body. Many of us believe certain foods are "bad" and others "good," when the truth is, it's how we use or perceive the food that is bad or good. This mentality generally focuses on what needs to be eliminated versus what is missing from our diets.

The relationship that we have with our food—as well as the way in which we talk to ourselves while we're eating—has a significant impact on how we digest and assimilate that food and what it does to our body and our state of mind.

ACTION ITEM

Jot down in your food journal what you are eating
and how you feel when you eat foods that
are supportive or destructive.

Four Paths

There are four distinct paths in yoga that can lead to lasting bliss and intentional living. Depending on your personality, you may choose one path over another, but each has the same goal.

In yoga's early days, people compared it to a tree, a living part of nature with complementary components that work together to thrive: roots, trunk, branches, leaves, blossoms, and so on. Yoga has many facets, just like life, but it always comes back to our ability to choose. This book didn't fall from the sky and land in your hands; you made the choice to read it and develop a Lean Consciousness that will better your health.

Raja Path—Yoga of Meditation

Raja is the path of self-control and mastery of your own mind. The person who chooses this path is able to become calm, still, and perfectly stable. Meditation and regular yoga and exercise, as well as clearing out clutter, will give you this control. When the mind is not restless, you are closer to self-awareness. To follow the path of raja, you must take a comprehensive approach—using the physical yoga practice to strengthen the body in order to sit in meditation, where the true union of body, mind, and spirit occurs. Raja yoga turns mental and physical energy into spiritual energy.

Instead of eating or drinking to channel feelings, the raja yogi turns to meditation to understand them, relax, and create a sense of peace.

Controlling the mind is possible; it just takes a certain level of awareness. One of the best ways to control is first to understand. Spending time every day to write down any negative feelings that plague you, especially feelings that may propel you to engage in unhealthy behaviors, will help you identify what these feelings are. Once you take time every day to immerse yourself in these feelings completely, you will understand them and yourself better. Sometimes the mere acknowledgment of a feeling allows it to dissipate. Once you have done this for a while, when the same feelings come up, acknowledge them and then allow them to release.

ACTION ITEM

Take ten to fifteen minutes a day to recognize
your feelings and feel them fully.

Karma Path—Yoga of Service and Action

Karma yoga focuses on the causes and effects of an individual's actions. It teaches how to live a life of spiritual or right action and selfless service. The true follower of the karma path acts without thought of gain or reward, which purifies the heart. To achieve this, it is helpful to keep your mind focused by repeating a mantra while engaged in any activity.

When we spend less time focusing on ourselves and more time projecting gratitude and service out to the world, our energy isn't bogged down. We are consciously serving others, spending our time for the greater good rather than dwelling on our problems. When we use our energy more positively, it overpowers those negative forces that hold us down.

Practice karma yoga by making choices that benefit others—volunteering, donating, and sharing your yoga practice with the less fortunate.

ACTION ITEM

Take time to delve deeply into your heart and find a cause or a group of individuals or animals that calls to your heart and may even make you weep with sorrow. Take time, on a monthly basis, to go and help this group. There is no better way to get yourself out of a downward spiral of food addiction than to give back to others with a higher purpose and beat the blues.

Jnana Path—Yoga of Knowledge

Jnana yoga seeks to bring out the knowledge in all of us through questioning, meditation, and contemplation. Jnana yoga includes the ability to differentiate between what is real/eternal and what is unreal/temporary.

Reading this book will give you jnana yoga. A well-rounded practice means educating yourself so that you know what's good for you and why. We all know that almonds are a great source of protein and fat, but what's a serving size? If you're eating handfuls at a time, you are defeating the purpose of your good intention. (Note: One serving of almonds is approximately a quarter cup—not an entire Costco bag.)

Get to know your supplements, food, diet, exercise, and yoga to create a tool chest to help lose weight.

ACTION ITEM

Take time daily to do ten to fifteen minutes of reading on nutrition, exercise, and other topics outlined in this book. Educate yourself on the workings of the body and the mind.
Make a plan to learn a new exercise every three months and study nutrition from a variety of sources. Keep a food and exercise journal with a notes section about how certain exercises and foods make you feel. Learn about your own body.

Bhakti Path—Yoga of Devotion

Opening the heart to the divine is the focus of bhakti, a mystical path of personal devotion. It is the path most followed in India, and it involves surrendering ourselves to the divine through prayer, worship, and ritual. Health is our most valuable asset. It's not healthy to smoke, to eat processed food, or to drink alcohol to excess. If we stay in a state of reverence, we are in a state of YogaLean. We must stay devoted to our body; it's what keeps us alive.

Chanting is an example of devotion. See chapter 7 on meditation to learn about the benefits of chanting to create a more positive world, for yourself and others.

ACTION ITEMS

To be in devotion—pray for health daily.
Sing or chant daily. Keep a photo of your best self in
perfect health or a reasonable role model you'd like to
look and feel like. Spend ten minutes a day in a state
of devotional gratitude for your good health.

———

Witness Consciousness Means Being Mindful and Aware

"Learn to listen to the body, and you are on your
way to witness consciousness."

The origin of the idea of Witness Consciousness and its practice is found in the Upanishads. The Upanishads are the sacred Hindu scriptures and are thought to be between five thousand and seven thousand years old.

To be a witness means watching and observing objectively. According to philosophy, whatever can be seen in the material world is not part of our essential nature but exists in a transient phase. Witness Consciousness, a yogic tool for self-development and self-understanding, is the unification muscle that finds a place beyond the body or the mind to allow us to become an observer of all the mind does: the judgments, the chatter, the distractions, the cravings, and the addiction. It's self-observation. Should I adjust my lifestyle to get more sleep, or should I get another Starbucks coffee?

When we use Witness Consciousness, it helps us to decipher the thousands of thoughts that race through our minds on a daily basis. The unification muscle is that place beyond the body that watches the mind and the mind and the body to recognize thoughts and insights.

The human condition by its very nature is associated with various emotions. Some emotions are positive, some are neutral, and some are destructive. Fear, anger, rage, and guilt undermine our peace of mind and our efforts to fulfill our potential. The practice of Witness Consciousness enables us to observe the origins of our emotions more clearly. It teaches us that our emotions are passing phenomena and not our true nature.

By developing watchfulness and an ability to observe yourself even in difficult circumstances, you can gradually weaken the roots of negativity and transform your mind. In fact, by reducing the power of negative emotions and uprooting them, Witness Consciousness can lead to an optimistic and positive frame of mind, which ultimately guides you away from unhealthy choices.

Those who practice mindfulness become more sensitive to their own natures as well as those of others. They develop a wonderful richness of the spirit and are helpful to their fellow human beings. Witness Consciousness helps them develop a non-judgmental and forgiving attitude toward themselves, which is a huge component of losing weight and staying healthy.

3
clearing space

..

"Only when we clean the window
do we really get to see inside and out."

by making the choice to become YogaLean, you are recognizing that you live in a situation, in a house, in a body that no longer suits you. You need to build a new and improved house by cleaning it from the inside out so that you are able to focus on your lean goals without all of the clutter. Let's say you're having a house makeover; prior to rebuilding the house, you need to clear the lot to set the stage for improvements. This is why it is important to clear your surrounding clutter before partaking of the YogaLean journey.

What is clutter? According to Dictionary.com, clutter is "a disorderly heap or assemblage" or "a state or condition of confusion"; as a verb, it means "to fill or litter with things in a disorderly matter."

Why do so many of us hold on to this thing called clutter—whether it be in a junk drawer, a disorganized closet or pantry, friends who give off negative energy, bad memories, fat stored in our body, and so on—when clutter is taking up vital space that can energize and fulfill us? It's because we have an emotional attachment to clutter and cannot let go. However, most of these possessions are merely hindering us from gaining Lean Consciousness and living a life of great intention. They are distracting us from feeling nourished and clean, and ultimately we need to redeem our space to start anew and become YogaLean.

We have the power to de-clutter, just like we have the power to say no to a side of french fries. Healthy living doesn't just mean diet and exercise. It also means limiting stressors that enter our lives and stick around, like unneeded stuff clogging up our space. Aside from a cleaner space, it can also mean turning off the TV and getting rid of the bad influences that we absorb when watching it, including stories we see on the news or food that entices us during commercials. Furthermore, it can mean getting rid of those people in our lives who hinder us and our goals.

Space! You need it, I need it, and your family needs it. We need space in our schedules to exercise, to practice yoga, to prepare healthy food, and to meditate. We need space to move around and not feel trapped. We need space to breathe and step away from the hustle and bustle of our day-to-day existence.

Yoga gives us both physical and mental space, and guess what, our environment is also in need of this space. Overeating is like hoarding food, cluttering our bodies with what we consume. Both are compulsive, excessive, and all-consuming. They also serve as self-protection, a means to feel better and avoid reality; this is why so many hoarders and overeaters live in secrecy and shame. When you become extremely attached to belongings or food, you begin to diminish, not only in self-respect but also in quality of life. De-cluttering our body and our space is important to fostering a sense of self-realization and respect.

There is a correlation between maintaining an orderly household and maintaining your ideal weight. As you begin your weight loss journey, I want you to start with a clean slate, clearing the clutter and taking back the energy that is lost and buried in your stuff. We often become a hostage to our possessions. Remember that all matter takes up space and energy. If things are in disarray, we may spend more time rummaging through them than on developing ourselves as people.

Since saucha (the niyama of cleanliness) is one of your goals, it needs to translate to your physical space as well as your body. De-cluttering is an emotional journey. It's not easy to surrender your possessions, but it's important to recognize (and be honest about) why you are holding on to certain things and if they are benefiting you or bogging you down.

When your physical environment is simplified and organized, you will have more mental and emotional space available to create and grow. When your kitchen reflects the same care and order you desire in your personal life, the time you spend there and the meals you produce will become capable of nourishing you in new ways. Taking time to make your kitchen a "sacred space" is an integral part of Yoga-Lean.

I spend an enormous amount of time thinking about the benefits of a clear space. And I've developed a little concept I like to call "zen-tervention™," meaning when we organize the physical aspects of our life, we are then better able to improve our fitness, food, finances, and lives.

When you have your personal zen-tervention, you will go through three steps: assessment, visualization, and clearing the decks. In each phase, you must embrace honesty and nonjudgment. With each item, assess why you are holding on to it and if it is serving you.

Assessment

Assess your living situation. Notice how you feel when you enter your home. Notice your immediate reaction beyond familiarity. Are there things that make you cringe, things you avoid dealing with, cleaning, or repairing?

Tomorrow morning, if you don't do this already, make your bed before leaving for work. When you come home and see that your bed is made, it will instantly change the dynamic of the room when you enter it. Is your sink filled with dishes? Clear the sink daily. Think about it: If you walk into a room after a stressful day and the first thing you see is a disorderly bed or overflowing sink, you will not feel orderly in your mind. Assess how your space makes you feel. Then pinpoint what is making it that way.

Often we fall into habits, so that even if things are dirty, broken, disorganized, or cluttered, we accept them because sometimes it's just too much work to fix them. If your house is organized on the surface, is there something that isn't as organized? Your closet? Do you have multiple junk drawers? How long has that banana been sitting on the bottom shelf of your freezer?

If you are having a difficult time seeing what is causing clutter, invite a friend, coach, or trainer to help you assess; someone who will support your journey and ask you, without judgment, if these things are serving you.

All objects are made of matter. Matter and objects take up energy; if you have too much stuff in the space, it will block your energy. These things could be sucking the life force right out of you, and you may not even know it. Your living space and in particular your kitchen should flow so that when you walk in, you will flow with it.

Visualize and Make a Reasonable Plan

"If you can see it, then you can be it."

—R. KELLY

Your home may never look like a spread from **Better Homes and Gardens,** **but it should** at the very least function. If you've ever seen the show *Hoarders,* you will notice that the dysfunction of the house is a reflection of the dysfunction of the person. It is our goal to clear that chaos one room at a time. First, make a plan for each room. For the purpose of YogaLean, I will guide you through your kitchen in hopes that your new clear space will open the doors to other rooms, closets, or even your car trunk.

Perhaps your kitchen needs a complete renovation from cabinets to counters to paint, or perhaps you simply need to purchase functional supplies that inspire you to cook. Your broken pans and dull knife aren't going to motivate you to whip up something great for dinner. But what will?

Create a plan or a list that shows you what you need or want to make your kitchen brighter and more functional. Even dramatic changes, like a mini-makeover, do not have to be costly.

Design a vision board of what your ideal kitchen would look like and what utensils and spices you need to cook seamlessly. In Part II of this book, I dive into clean eating and foods that will aid your body and mind. Make a list of those foods so that you can fill your pantry, fridge, and freezer with them.

Make a list of the foods that make you feel groggy or that you know are bad for you—your secret candy stash, the junk food that you find yourself aimlessly gnawing on in moments of despair, the indulgent Dove Bars. With each item, think about what it's contributing to the good of your body.

Clear the Decks

In order to get and stay lean, we must continuously be able to let go of things that are not working. Remember that YogaLean is a combination of changing your body and your life. If you live in a distressed, unclean environment, your body will soon reflect that. Set an example for yourself. Sentimentality will keep you stuck in the past. To be lean is to let go—again and again—and to stay in the present moment.

Commit yourself to this project by blocking off a Saturday or Sunday or even taking a day off of work. If you're open to it, grab a friend or two to help out. Make sure to have some great music and some good tea or coffee for extra energy. Wear your favorite workout clothes, or put on the things that make you feel your best, whether that's light makeup, a dab of perfume, or your favorite scarf. Make yourself excited, like it's an event.

Start clearing the decks. Take everything out of your kitchen—and I do mean everything. Get three large cardboard boxes and label them "Toss," "Donate," and "Keep." Then clear out all the cabinets, counters, and shelves as well as the refrigerator.

This is an important step toward developing Lean Consciousness and is part of the letting-go process. Things look different when they are clear. Once everything is out of the space, reassess what you need and what is important to your kitchen.

Toss anything that is old, broken, or expired or that you have not used in the past year or no longer serves a purpose—for instance, your old Fry Daddy deep fryer. Go through your kitchen cabinets, fridge, and freezer—toss or donate any food that contains white flour, sugar, hydrogenated corn syrup, or trans fats. Throw out any sauces, spices, dressings, or condiments that are expired or more than six months old. *Fresh* is everything. Get rid of anything that is not helping you move in the right direction. You are either moving toward your goals or away from them. If you feel uncomfortable throwing something out and you feel it's appropriate to donate it to a charitable organization, then feel free to do so.

Keep items, tools, gadgets, whole grains, and other goods that will help you on your YogaLean mission to live a healthier, better you!

Clean! Use new sponges—old ones carry bacteria that can cause sickness. Always have clean sponges around! While the cabinets, pantry, drawers, and fridge are empty, clean them . . . yourself! If you do it, not only are you burning extra calories, but you are also literally putting your energy into the space to make it cleaner.

Fill a spray bottle with a natural cleaning solution of white vinegar, the juice of half a lemon, and water. Start spritzin' and get your kitchen cabinets, countertops, floors, and refrigerator fully and completely clean. Get on your knees and deep clean, vacuum, dust, mop, scrub, and soak. Freshen up your space. If you have the energy, put on a new coat of paint or sand/refinish your cabinets, or simply line your cupboards with organic paper or natural sisal lining for freshness, cleanliness, and beauty.

Shop and Restock

In order to make an exquisite meal, you need a good knife; a pot, pan, or baking dish; a mixing bowl; and typically a wooden spoon. If your knife is dull, either buy a new one or get it sharpened. If your bowls and plates are chipped, ask yourself why you're eating off of them. It can be very inexpensive to replace dishes if you do a minute of research or go to a restaurant supply store, Target, Overstock.com, Cooking.com, or Home Goods. Here are some YogaLean kitchen basics:

- Paring knife
- Butcher's knife

- Dishes that are not chipped
- Two cutting boards (one for meats, one for produce)
- Small blender for smoothies
- Food processor (if you don't like cutting)
- Smaller plates (these will promote smaller portions)
- Skillet
- Soup pot
- Glass baking dish

See my recommendations for a well-stocked pantry in the recipe chapter.

Once your kitchen is done, you may feel so good that you decide to take on one room at a time until the entire house is fresh and bright. When the objects in your space take up less energy and attention, you can focus on achieving your goals in health. As you begin to toss and donate your belongings, you will become lighter. This will move you toward a deeper state of Lean Consciousness.

ACTION ITEM

Pick one thing to clear, organize, or dispose of
every day for forty days.

4
the power of breath

..

"Make your breath bigger
than your physical body."

b reath is life. I've briefly touched on prānāyāma, an essential component
of the Eight Limbs of YogaLean, and now I want to dive deep into its importance to our health and clearing space. Learning how to connect the
limbs through breath, exercise, clean eating, and meditation will create open space
in your lungs and body.

While yoga practitioners have used breathing practices for thousands of years,
scientists in the Western world have only recently recognized that deep, controlled
breathing has a direct correlation with improved health. With breath and meditation, we are able to reduce stress, which as we all know is linked to a number of serious health conditions, including high blood pressure, heart disease, depression, and
sometimes weight gain. Learning how to breathe deeply both on and off our mats
can clear the loud noise stored in our brains and reduce or even eliminate a majority
of the symptoms triggered by stress.

In *The Yoga of Breath,* Richard Rosen lists some of the reported physical, psychological, and spiritual benefits of practicing prānāyāma and also describes how it can "stoke the gastric fire, which improves digestion and speeds elimination of wastes from the body, and appease thirst and hunger so you won't be distracted by these cravings during practice; open the sinuses to allow more air into the body; purify both the gross and subtle energy systems of the body; and cure many diseases and conditions, including nervous disorders, indigestion, cough, and fever."

When taking time to breathe, and I'm talking intentional breath, we allow ourselves to live in the moment, to slow down, to evaluate impulse decisions, and to connect with Lean Consciousness during moments of despair. Rather than devouring a box of Oreos because you feel bad or eating quickly because that's what you're used to, breathing will bring you back to your journey and allow you to feel what you're feeling instead of eating it.

The practice of prānāyāma (breathing), according to the Yoga Sutras, also helps with the limbs of dhāranā (concentration), dhyāna (meditation), and samādhi (physical connection or oneness). Breath lies at the core of these limbs and not only fuels all of our bodily functions but also aids in mental clarity and focus.

As you may recall, the first niyama, saucha, is the practice of cleanliness and purification. Prior to incorporating a breathing technique into your day, you must first clear your passageway for your breath's life force (prana) to function unobstructed. And of course, in order to partake in certain breathing techniques, it's important to ensure your nasal passages are also "de-cluttered."

Use a Neti Pot to Clear Your Nadis for Prānāyāma

Jala neti is the act of cleansing the nasal passages with water. Neti is becoming more widespread in doctor's offices, hospitals, Ayurvedic clinics, and yoga therapy programs and as an accessible at-home treatment for runny noses, allergies, sinus problems, and even headaches. It is a ritual with a distinguished pedigree, described in ancient Sanskrit texts on yoga and Ayurveda. In these medical and metaphysical works, neti is suggested for everything from chronic stuffy noses to the development of intuition, insight, and clear perception. Neti can be an important ritual for people who live in polluted environments or work in professions where they are subjected to smog, dust, dirt, or other irritants. While neti is often suggested after surgery, check with your healthcare provider before starting a neti practice if you have had recent surgery or have other health considerations.

How to Practice Neti

Neti involves rinsing the nasal passages with salt water using a **neti pot**, which resembles a small watering can with a small spout to set inside the nostril.

Dr. Carrie Demers, who practices at the Himalayan Institute's Total Health Center in Honesdale, Pennsylvania, suggests using filtered water and a quarter-teaspoon of salt for a standard size pot. Sometimes it can be helpful to taste the solution, which should taste like tears and not the ocean. Too much or too little salt can feel uncomfortable.

Breathing Practices

*Once you've cleared your nasal passages, you are set to begin your breathing. We prac-*tice the following techniques in YogaFit; these are great for beginners who are learning to understand their breath and becoming one with it.

Three-Part Breath—The Complete Breath

This is the simplest and most rewarding of all yogic breathing exercises. It is both purifying and energizing and, if done slowly and evenly, can produce a sense of serenity and balance. Breathing in and out to nearly the full vital capacity a few times can markedly increase blood oxygen levels and decrease carbon dioxide. This is a great awareness tool for beginners to realize the potential depth of their breath and the capacity of their lungs.

There is a therapeutic effect of the three-part breath—our basic yogic breath—it calms the nervous system and increases delivery of prana. In *Perfect Breathing*, Al Lee and Don Campbell write, "Breath awareness means exactly what it says—being aware of or observing the quality of your breath, whether it is shallow or deep, long or short, easy or labored, smooth or uneven. Conscious breathing, often referred to as controlled breathing, intentional breathing, and mindful breathing, refers to breathing with purpose. Though there may be subtle differences in the meanings of these terms, they all imply breathing to achieve a result of some kind, whatever it may be, as opposed to the passive act of breath awareness."

The "three parts" are the abdomen, diaphragm, and chest. During three-part breath, first you completely fill your lungs with air, as though you are breathing into your belly, ribcage, and upper chest. Then you exhale completely, reversing the flow.

Practice:

1. When you inhale, guide the air to the bottom of the lungs, then fill the ribcage followed by the chest.
2. When you exhale, relax the chest and let out the air naturally; then relax the ribcage and, finally, complete the exhale with the air from the belly.
3. Begin with ease, and gradually, let the breath deepen.
4. At the top of the inhale, the chest should lift up gently. At the bottom of the exhale, the abdomen should be all the way in.
5. Start with five minutes.

Alternate Nostril Breathing

It is said in Ayurveda and in the therapeutic yoga tradition that alternate nostril breathing can be helpful for equalizing the activity in the right and left hemispheres of the brain; it can relax the nervous system and calm the mind. In general, when we do alternate nostril breathing, we literally switch which nostril we breathe in and out of in a rhythmic pattern. Not everyone knows that the movement of our breath naturally switches from one nostril to the other approximately every 90 to 120 minutes. For example, breath flowing through the right nostril is more stimulating, while breath moving through the left nostril is more quieting or sedating.

Breathing through one nostril stimulates the flow of energy through the opposite or contralateral side of the brain, as the nadis (the different channels in which the energies of the subtle body flow to connect the chakras, which are the body's points of intensity) crisscross through the body. Modern studies, including one published in 2004 in the journal *Neurological Science,* demonstrate through the use of modern physiological testing that breathing through one nostril not only activates the movement of prana through the nadis but also impacts the electrical and metabolic activity in the contralateral hemisphere of the brain. This not only has important implications for our consciousness and our state of mind, it also reinforces the therapeutic benefit of prānāyāma practice.

To alternate between the two nostrils encourages equanimity, clarity of thought, a feeling of being centered, and even an experience of mental and subtle body purification. The Sanskrit name for this breath, *nadi shodhana*, speaks to this, because it translates to "cleansing the nadis," which allows us to experience greater balance. This breath practice helps to calm the mind, to encourage mental focus, and to prepare the mind and physical and subtle bodies for other types of practices.

Alternate nostril breathing is a practice that can be done anytime by anybody. One of its greatest benefits is to encourage the parasympathetic nervous system, reducing our body's experience of stress, something we all need. While we might not want to practice this while at a stoplight or sitting in a traffic jam, other times, like during a break in the workday, before getting the kids ready for school, or at the end of the day, can be perfect for practicing alternate nostril breathing. According to Siva Samhita, an ancient Sanskrit text on yoga, yogis who practice purification of the nadis "sit up straight, are fragrant, are beautiful, and are a receptacle for the nectar of the gods."

According to Ayurveda and yogic theory, some activities actually work better when one nostril is more active. For example, after meals, Ayurveda suggests that if one is going to lie down, lie down on the left side, because then the right nostril is more active; breathing through the right nostril is more heating and helps to stimulate digestion. On the other hand, if someone has trouble falling asleep, lying down on the right side can be beneficial for promoting sound sleep, because then the left nostril is more active, and this is the cooling side of the body, which allows for a greater degree of calm and ease.

Sometimes, due to congestion or other factors, the breath getting stuck in one nostril can affect our state of mind; engaging in a breathing practice can create a shift in physical, mental, or emotional expression. The therapeutic use of a neti pot can also be helpful for making sure that the breath, and therefore the prana, can move easily between the right and left nostrils, and the ida and pingala nadis, which address the female and male energies.

RIGHT (SOLAR)—NOSTRIL BREATH (SURYA BHEDANA)

LEFT (LUNAR)—NOSTRIL BREATH (CHANDRA BHEDANA)

The physical, mental, emotional, and spiritual effects of right and left nostril breathing relate to the movement of the prana through the nadis from the point of view of yogic anatomy and physiology and to the activity of the nervous system from the point of view of Western anatomy and physiology. When we examine both points of view, we see the synergy between the seemingly disparate approaches. Right nostril breath is the warming or stimulating breath used to increase energy or alertness, and the left nostril has the opposite effects. These breaths can be used to balance the doshas, the three different body types—which we will learn more about later—when necessary. The Hatha Yoga Pradipika, a Sanskrit yoga manual that focuses on hatha, advises against the use of chandra bhedana unless you are being advised by a guru, due to the possibility of lowering the energy too much.

To practice alternate nostril breathing, it is traditional to use your right hand, specifically the thumb and ring finger, to close one nostril gently, allowing yourself to breathe through the other.

Sometimes people with a deviated septum or other abnormalities, or malformations such as polyps in the nose or other issues, may have difficulties with alternate nostril breathing.

Practice:

1. Find a comfortable seated position with your spine straight and upright.
2. Use your thumb to seal your right nostril gently so that you can begin by exhaling through your left nostril as long as it is comfortable.
3. Then inhale through your left nostril as long as it is comfortable.
4. Switch the position of your right hand by gently sealing your left nostril.
5. Exhale through your right nostril and then inhale through your right nostril.
6. This represents one round or sequence of alternate nostril breathing; depending on your capacity, repeat ten times (or practice for several minutes).
7. This practice can help center the mind before a busy day, work, or an exam. It also creates a state of calm for an enjoyable session of meditation.

Breath of Fire

Breath of fire (kapālabhātī) uses deep, rapid breath cycles to warm your body and to increase your energy. Traditionally, the breath of fire is not a prāṇāyāma technique but rather a kriyā, or cleansing, practice. Many of the toxins in your body are released during your exhale, which is the focus here. Practice it during Mountains 1 and 3, which we'll address in chapter 6. Some of the effects: it energizes and activates the right side of your pranic system (your energy flow), stimulates your nervous system, and cleanses your respiratory system.

Practice:

1. Find a comfortable seated or reclining position.
2. Keeping your mouth closed, begin inhaling through your nose.
3. Exhale half the air out of your lungs to a point somewhere between exhale and inhale.
4. Your exhale should be quick and sharp, contracting your abdominal muscles. In this exercise, exhalations are short, vigorous, and active; inhalations are light and passive.
5. Continue this rhythmic pattern for twenty to twenty-five breaths. Repeat two to five rounds, finishing with a deep three-part breath.

Clearing the Body

In addition to eating healthy on a consistent basis, people often turn to different forms of cleansing to flush the body of toxins, detoxify, and "start anew." Juicing, cleanses, or colonics are different and have precautions that are well worth discussing with your doctor before proceeding.

Juicing and Cleanses

The popularity of juice cleanses has risen dramatically recently with claims that they cure the common cold, detoxify the body, and lead to clarity and energy. While juicing or cleansing, a person will limit him- or herself to a liquid diet—vegetable or fruit juice, water, or the "master cleanse" of cayenne/honey/lemon, to name a few—for several days or weeks to restart the body from a clean state.

I am a fan of taking a periodic day or two off food and just drinking water and juices to get your digestive fire, your agni, back up. I find this very helpful if I have digestive issues, which I often do when traveling.

However, restricting your weekly intake to juices will prevent you from consuming the fat, protein, and carbs you need to maintain physical and cognitive functioning. Not only that, but when fruits and vegetables are pressed through a juicer, they are stripped of their fiber, which is a key component for weight loss. So I suggest limiting your cleanse time unless you are supervised, by a health center like We Care Holistic Health Center in Desert Hot Springs, California, or a naturopath doctor.

I also suggest going for a vegetable blend and avoiding pure fruit juices to limit your sugar intake.

Colonics

Colon cleansing is typically prescribed by doctors as a form of preparation for certain medical procedures, including colonoscopies. However, according to the Mayo Clinic, colon cleansing is not recommended to detoxify, because your digestive system and bowel naturally eliminate waste material and bacteria without the aid of colon cleansing.

It is believed, with little evidence, that toxins from your gastrointestinal tract can cause a variety of health problems, such as arthritis, allergies, and asthma, and that colon cleansing will rid the body of those toxins, creating an improved health and immune system.

Stomach Pumping (*Agni Saur Dhauti*)

Agni saur dhauti, the Sanskrit name of the important practice of stomach pumping, means "to wash the digestive fire." It is a powerful heating and cleansing practice. While this can be done every day (or nearly every day), only do so on an empty stomach. Some contraindications for this practice include pregnancy, ulcers, inflammatory bowel conditions, uncontrolled high blood pressure, and glaucoma.

Begin as you would start an abdominal lift: standing, knees bent, and leaning forward. (See Appendix B.) When you have the breath held out and the abdominal muscles pulled in, first release the muscles (without changing the breath) and then pull them back in as far as possible. Repeat this pumping action in and out as long as you can comfortably hold the breath out. Before you breathe in, feel all of the muscles completely relax. Repeat this for a few rounds if it feels good.

This technique helps strengthen digestive fire to stimulate early-morning appetite (so we can benefit from a good breakfast); to tone the abdominal muscles, including the muscles of the organs; and to reduce bloating, constipation, and abdominal discomfort.

ACTION ITEM

Sit for ten minutes twice a day and do deep three-part abdominal breathing. Download the YogaLean app, which will provide you with guided meditation.

5
understanding body type

..

"Every body is a yoga body."

When we look at the people around us, we see different shapes and sizes. This diversity represents the expression of the unique bodies we all possess, categorizing us as true individuals. Accepting and understanding your body will help you on the road to YogaLean.

Remembering the essence of YogaFit—letting go of judgment, expectation, and competition; breathing, feeling, listening to our body—connects us to the process of understanding our personal body type. By observing ourselves, by taking action based on our individuality, and by listening to our bodies, we have the opportunity to make choices that will benefit us as individuals.

There are many ways to categorize body type, all based on observation of patterns. Here I use the terminology of Ayurveda, which provides a framework to identify these patterns and enhance our health and well-being based on what our body needs.

Three Body Types

Ayurveda and yoga identify or categorize three general body types or "doshas"—vata, pitta, and kapha. Identifying each of the three body types on their own, with their sets of tendencies, strengths, and challenges, is illuminating. We may wonder why we feel sleepy every afternoon at 4 P.M., why we wake up at 3 A.M., or why we crave sweets or salty chips. While everyone is different, knowing the general habits of our body type can help us master the tools and practices that allow our bodies to thrive; these include recipes, exercise regimens, daily routines, and ongoing remedies.

- VATA is the principle of space, air, and movement. It governs all movement in the body. Anything related to vata is light, airy, spacious, expansive, changeable, movable, dry, cold, and erratic.
- PITTA is the principle of fire. It governs all digestion and transformation in the body. Anything related to pitta is hot, has the quality of rising upward, and is bright and intense.
- KAPHA is the principle of stability, water, and earth. It governs all structure, strength, and stamina. Anything related to kapha is slow, steady, heavy, dull, slow to move or change, wet, damp, dense, and cold.

While there are three distinct categories in the Ayurvedic system, one of the things that makes this different than other body type systems (such as blood type or endomorph/ectomorph/mesomorph) is that we are each a *combination* of vata, pitta, and kapha. We can describe people as being predominantly vata, pitta, or kapha. For instance, we may see in ourselves or other people a tendency toward being airy and irregular, fiery and intense, or solid and slow.

However, we all possess some measure of all three doshas: We move (vata); we digest (pitta); we have structure (kapha).

And we are not necessarily simply one type. It is not so easy to just say, "I'm a vata." You may have certain tendencies that clearly fall into one category or another, but most of us demonstrate all three tendencies in varying proportions.

Sometimes one dosha is so dominant in someone that this is all we see, like a thin, slight, spacy, vata-predominant person. Alternatively, a person may have one dosha with a dominant influence and another not far behind, such as an intense pitta who also has a lot of physical substance and even stubbornness (kapha). Yet another option is for two doshas to be equally influential, so someone might be intense and erratic. More rarely, some people are a combination of all three doshas equally.

This unique proportion gives each of us an individual nature, one that we can celebrate when we look in the mirror. Seeing a wide range of bodies that are all beautiful and healthy in different shapes, sizes, and patterns reminds us of the essence of YogaFit and why we need to let go of judgment, competition, and expectation.

Understanding these qualities can provide the information that allows us to showcase our strengths and support our challenges rather than fight against our physiology. Embracing your individuality and letting go of competition will reinforce your ability to maintain a body that is YogaLean.

For more information on each of the doshas, check out appendix A.

Assess Your Body Type

BODY TYPE QUIZ

Whenever you take a body type quiz, there are a few important points to keep in mind. First, take note of what feels true for you over the long term (not just how you feel today, the day you're taking the quiz). Second, this is an open book test—it's okay to ask your trusted friends and loved ones for their honest opinion when you are trying to assess yourself. Third, have compassion for yourself and see yourself as you are, not who you'd like to be or wish you were. Also, when answering the questions, think about other members of your family as a point of comparison, since every trait is on a continuum.

It can sometimes be helpful to take more than one quiz. A quick search of dosha quizzes on the Internet reveals a number of different online tests. The Chopra Center, Dr. Oz, the Ayurvedic Institute, and Banyan Botanicals are just a few of the websites offering ways for you to evaluate yourself online.

The important thing to note is that you're not looking for absolute measurements but rather a general sense of proportions. Are you predominantly pitta? Mostly vata? Do you have a tendency toward kapha? It's okay to circle more than one answer if you're on the fence, since the exact number isn't important.

One way to measure your frame is to take one hand and wrap your fingers around your opposite wrist. If your thumb overlaps your middle finger, you have a small frame. If they touch, you likely have a medium frame. If they barely or do not touch, you likely have a large frame.

ACTION ITEM

Try to fit yourself in to some of these categories to start to understand your body type in a general way.

VATA	PITTA	KAPHA
slender frame	medium frame	large frame, dense bone structure
slender hips/shoulders	hourglass figure, medium hips/shoulders	broad shoulders
slender muscles	defined muscles, builds easily	abundance of natural insulation, but pattern can shift with training
dry skin/hair/nails	tendency toward oily skin	soft, thick skin
tendency to be petite or tall	balanced proportions	balanced proportions, but dense joints
joints often crack or pop	joints can be inflamed	dense/thick, often short fingers/toes
arms/legs short or long	medium proportions	high stamina
low stamina	medium stamina	

VATA	PITTA	KAPHA
Skin	Skin	Skin
tans easily dry cold loves the sun chapped lips/skin (esp. feet) low sweat	burns easily, freckles oily warm or hot irritated by sun breaks out easily sweats easily	pale, tans slowly thick, soft cool, can be clammy warmed by the sun but sensitive soft sweats moderately
Nails	Nails	Nails
brittle, short	oily/yellowish	thick/grow quickly
Teeth	Teeth	Teeth
small/easily crooked	medium/yellowish	large/white/healthy
Gums	Gums	Gums
receding	prone to inflammation	healthy/pink
Hair	Hair	Hair
thin, dry prone to flaky scalp	oily, thick, prematurely gray breakout prone	thick, lots of hair thick skin under hair
Weight Gain/Loss Tendencies	Weight Gain/Loss Tendencies	Weight Gain/Loss Tendencies
loses weight easily weight can fluctuate hard to keep weight on	generally maintains average weight gains and loses	gains weight easily weight creeps upward hard to take weight off
Weight Gain Patterns	Weight Gain Patterns	Weight Gain Patterns

gain: hips/thighs/butt	gain: belly, midsection (apple),
	    arms/entire body
		gain: shoulders, chest (pear),
		    arms/entire body

VATA	PITTA	KAPHA
Cravings and Eating Patterns*	Cravings and Eating Patterns*	Cravings and Eating Patterns*
craves salty, crunchy tendency to skip meals small appetite fasting is challenging awakens depleted when meals are skipped, feels spacy/tired/fatigued	craves sweet, liquids frequently hungry loves to eat needs fluids regularly awakens physically hungry when meals are skipped, feels angry/frustrated/impatient	craves comfort foods "why skip a meal?" tendency to overeat can skip meals without ill effect hunger takes time to build up when meals are skipped, feels desolate
Mental/Psychological	Mental/Psychological	Mental/Psychological
auditory prone to anxiety/fear, imagination	visual prone to anger/impatience, implementation	feeling prone to stubbornness/resistance, stability
Memory	Memory	Memory
easy to remember easy to forget quick to anger resistant to habit/routine	easy to remember slow to forget moderate anger but intense good planner	takes time to sink in doesn't forget slow to anger but hangs on tendency toward stagnation
Sleep Patterns	Sleep Patterns	Sleep Patterns
trouble falling/staying asleep restless legs or body active mind	rise of energy around midnight excess heat/inflammation active mind	sleeps deeply and easily heaviness when sleeping can be slow
Dreams	Dreams	Dreams
flying anxious, worrying	adventure, violence passionate	water calm, peaceful
Menstrual Cycle	Menstrual Cycle	Menstrual Cycle
irregular, cramping	regular, heavy bleeding	regular, water retention

* While everyone craves sweets since they calm us when we're under stress, there are different patterns that can reveal more about body type.

VATA	PITTA	KAPHA
Digestion	Digestion	Digestion
irregular tendency to constipation or alternate constipation and diarrhea cramps easily sensitive to foods	intense regular tendency to loose stools steady can digest anything	slow sometimes sluggish steady

Takeaways

HOW TO KEEP VATA BALANCED

If your constitution is predominantly vata or characterized by an abundance of the energy of air, space, and lightness, then gaining weight may actually be challenging. You're the one who can eat anything, and your friends always say how lucky you are, but you know how frustrating it is to feel so light. If this energetic quality is out of balance, one of the ways that it can manifest is in depletion.

But just because you have trouble gaining weight doesn't mean that you are healthy or truly maintaining Lean Consciousness. Slender is not the same as balanced. Maintaining a slight frame can be easy until it isn't, until the metabolic, energetic, or emotional imbalances can throw off your usual set point.

Many things that have the qualities of vata increase that energetic quality and run the risk of throwing us out of balance. The challenge of this is that a large number of these are part and parcel of our everyday life. And in fact, the teachings of Ayurveda suggest that no matter what our basic body type or constitution is, we all have to be aware of the tendency for the light, airy, erratic, movable vata dosha (see appendix A) to be out of balance.

Since the energetic pattern of the vata dosha is airy and spacious, qualities, substances, and activities with this same energetic pattern increase vata. Too much of an increase of any of these qualities can lead to imbalance.

Eat at regular times (even eating one meal a day, such as breakfast, at a consistent time).

Make sure to eat some light protein or something substantial at each meal. Avoid or reduce iced water and ice-cold food and drinks—cold increases the constriction and the imbalance of the vata dosha.

Have something warm with each meal, such as a cup of hot water with lemon, room-temperature water, hot herbal tea, hot soup or miso, or hot cereal.

Make sure to take in enough salts and electrolytes. Vata-type people often crave salt because it is calming and grounding.

Be careful of caffeine and other stimulants; use them judiciously. Caffeine and stimulants can create imbalance in the nervous system, exaggerating the tendencies of the energy of the vata dosha to be anxious, nervous, and irritable, to have trouble sleeping, or to experience the negative effects of an increased stress response.

GENERAL TIPS

- Soak in hot baths, Jacuzzi, hot springs, or warm water
- Listen to music you love
- Massage, including gentle self-massage
- Forward folds
- Legs up against wall
- Create as much healthy routine as possible
- Ensure that physical activity is both activating and restorative
- Engage in regular stretching as part of a routine
- Create sleep rituals before bed to promote sound sleep
- Use nose oils
- Eat ashwagandha and chavyanprash (see chapter 10)

HOW TO KEEP PITTA BALANCED

Since the pitta body type has a tendency for intensity, make sure to cultivate a sense of calm and to employ numerous stress reduction techniques to maintain the type of balance needed to prevent high cortisol levels from taking hold and contributing to weight gain.

One of the characteristics of the pitta dosha is a strong digestive fire. Carry snacks and make sure to eat meals at regular times. Skipping meals or feeling hungry can increase the grouchy factor, aggravating the body's stress response and increasing the risk of anger and irritation flaring up.

Maintaining balance for pitta isn't just about keeping the body YogaLean, it's also about keeping the mind calm, cool, and collected. This starts with eating meals regularly to keep the mind clear—and choosing anti-inflammatory foods such as dark green leafy vegetables, whole grains, and lean and vegetarian proteins. Pitta people should also watch out for excessive caffeine intake, since caffeine increases cortisol levels in the body and can increase the risk of cortisol weight gain.

People with a lot of pitta tendencies have a sweet tooth and often crave sweets to calm themselves down. Choosing healthy whole-grain complex carbohydrates such as brown rice, quinoa, and even sweet potatoes can support the need for sweet foods that are actually nourishing and don't run the risk of throwing you further out of balance.

Listening to music that you love is a good way to soothe the mind and reduce stress. Getting a good night's sleep is also one of the best ways to reset the intense pitta mind.

GENERAL TIPS

- Walk by the ocean, rivers, streams, or other bodies of water
- Inversions
- Twists
- Sweat out all the stress and tension and then incorporate a soothing savasana practice, a yoga technique where you lie on your back with your arms and legs spread at about 45 degrees, close your eyes, and take long, deep breaths
- Listen to music that helps you relieve stress
- Use mantras or positive affirmations to help you achieve goals or direct an active mind
- Regular meditation practice
- Yoga sequences that are challenging yet restorative
- Regular sleep practices

- Cooling foods such as cucumber, coconut, dark green leafy vegetables
- Turmeric
- Triphala (see chapter 10)
- Swimming as exercise to cool off the body
- When running or working out, choose early morning or evening hours when the sun is less intense
- Weight training to balance hormone levels and reduce stress and burn off any internal aggression
- Aromatherapy oils including lavender, rose, geranium, sandalwood, shatavari

HOW TO KEEP KAPHA BALANCED

Since kapha has a tendency to be heavy, stagnant, slow, and sluggish, maintaining balance involves creating more internal heat, stimulation, and strength. People with a lot of kapha tendencies may have a love of comfort and are sometimes couch potatoes, but they are the ones who most need healthy, strong, and consistent movement in their lives. Get up and get moving! Sweat and heat it up in every area of your life. Try new things, go outside, find a workout buddy, and make an appointment to go to the gym or to yoga together, walk as much as possible and spice up your diet.

Trade iced drinks for hot ones. Instead of a tall glass of iced water, drink hot water with lemon, lime, or ginger.

People with a lot of kapha tendencies sleep easily and well, but be careful of oversleeping, sleeping in, or taking too many naps in the afternoon. Set the alarm to wake up before sunrise and go outside and enjoy the early-morning hours.

Be careful of the tendency to love comfort foods—these are the ones that can weigh you down.

According to the teachings of Ayurveda, people with a lot of kapha tendencies are the ones who can best tolerate caffeine and might even benefit from the lift, particularly from something like green tea (rather than a latte with a lot of heavy milk).

Make sure to keep your schedule active and full of stimulation so as not to slide into complacency. In every way, think heat and stimulate.

GENERAL TIPS

- Give yourself a good sweat at least once a day through yoga (YogaFit Sweat will really get you going), cardio, weight training, walking as often as possible, or even using a sauna
- Digestive practices including agni saur dhauti and nauli (see appendix B)
- Include back bends in your practice to improve circulation and remove stagnation around the upper chest and heart
- Step outside and spend as much time in the sun as possible
- Drink hot water with lemon first thing in the morning to stimulate digestion, elimination, and detoxification, and ginger tea and peppermint with meals to stimulate the digestive fire
- Add hot, pungent spices to meals to stimulate digestion and metabolism, including cayenne, jalapeno, ginger, black pepper, and horseradish
- Eat light, especially at night, and make vegetables the largest part of the plate, substituting savory for sweet in meals—even try starting the day with a savory rather than sweet breakfast
- Incorporate dry brushing into your daily routine to stimulate lymphatic circulation
- Give yourself a massage on a weekly basis with stimulating oil blends that include uplifting scents like rosemary or eucalyptus to encourage good overall circulation
- Triphala (see chapter 10)
- Heating breath practices such as breath of fire; since kapha needs heat and stimulation in order not to stagnate, the overall prescription is more fire
- Music that has a drumbeat or a stimulating effect

How to Balance Life Depending on Time of Day and Season

The energies that affect our bodies also cycle through the day. When we understand how they cycle, it can give us information about how to organize our daily routine to support Lean Consciousness.

CYCLES OF THE DOSHAS THROUGH THE DAY

6:00 a.m.–10:00 a.m.	Kapha predominates (earth/water)
10:00 a.m.–2:00 p.m.	Pitta predominates (fire)
2:00 p.m.–6:00 p.m.	Vata predominates (air/space)
6:00 p.m.–10:00 p.m.	Kapha predominates (earth/water)
10:00 p.m.–2:00 a.m.	Pitta predominates (fire)
2:00 a.m.–6:00 a.m.	Vata predominates (air/space)

6:00 a.m.–10:00 a.m.   Kapha Predominates (earth/water)

Ayurvedic daily routine suggests waking up and getting out of bed before 6 A.M.—before the transition to the kapha time of day. When we sleep much past 6 A.M., it is as though we are trying to rouse ourselves from underneath the heavy wet blanket of the kapha dosha. The benefit, though, of this kapha time of the morning is that it is a time of great strength and stamina. It can be one of the best and most productive times of day, since we are experiencing energetic support. Doing something before breakfast to stimulate digestive fire (practices), drinking hot water with lemon to detoxify and strengthen digestion, or having ginger or peppermint tea—these are powerful ways to support digesting breakfast with ease.

10:00 a.m.–2:00 p.m.   Pitta Predominates (fire)

According to this system, pitta represents the energy of fire, transformation, and digestion. For this reason, Ayurveda strongly recommends that we eat our largest and most substantial meal at lunchtime, when we have the support of a strong digestive fire to assimilate the nutrients fully. Ayurveda does believe that breakfast is important to jumpstart the day, just as we know that eating breakfast on a consistent basis is necessary for metabolic consistency and for maintenance of the YogaLean lifestyle.

2:00 p.m.–6:00 p.m.   Vata Predominates (air/space)

Lunch is also important to give us the strength and clarity to maintain consistent energy through the afternoon. The mid-afternoon time is characterized by a prevalence of the airy vata dosha. How many times have we felt an energetic crash in the middle of the afternoon? This is because of a natural cycle. Just as the sun rises and sets, so too the doshas cycle.

During the vata cycle, we more likely feel spacy, airy, light, empty, tired, and maybe even anxious. In some cultures, this is siesta time. Instead of trying to pull up our energy, we should allow ourselves to relax and socialize and chat and enjoy the spaciness. But if we need to be productive at work, we have to be careful of a tendency to turn to stimulants and sugar to boost our energy, particularly if we have not had a lunch that supports our energetic needs. The mid-afternoon sugar and stimulant break can wreak havoc with our plan for living YogaLean. This is because the stimulants that raise cortisol and increase the body's stress response can lead to greater deposits of abdominal fat. The sugar rush interferes with metabolic consistency, which helps maintain regular blood sugar levels and support a healthy weight.

6:00 p.m.–10:00 p.m.   Kapha Predominates (earth/water)

We may finally feel a sense of relief around 6 P.M. That's because the rug that was pulled out from under us during the empty vata time of day has been returned to its rightful place. We feel stronger, more settled, ready for family time or workouts. This is a good time of day for us to enjoy the positive qualities of the kapha dosha: love, connection, ease, and steadiness.

According to Ayurveda, a healthy routine includes getting ready for bed and allowing the body to wind down during this time of day. While we can work out in the evening to prepare for sleep, it is also true that the later the evening hours progress, the more we benefit from activities that are restorative, rejuvenating, and calming to the nervous system. Meditation, restorative yoga practices, and relaxation techniques all help us to benefit from the hours we will be asleep.

10:00 p.m.–2:00 a.m.   Pitta Predominates (fire)

Since the next pitta, or fire-dominant, time of day begins at 10 P.M., Ayurveda suggests being in bed and falling asleep as close to 10 P.M. as possible. Have you ever experienced a second wind or a rise in energy after 10 P.M.? That's because the fire in our body has risen. While we may be tempted to use this surge of energy to clean the house, catch up with our friends on Facebook, or return the day's emails, save those midnight energy marathons for the times you really need them. This energy of fire and digestion is also responsible for the body's repair mechanisms. You may have heard that the hours before midnight are some of our most important hours of sleep. This is why. The body also produces growth hormones at this time of night, during the stages of deep sleep.

2:00 a.m.–6:00 a.m.   Vata Predominates (air/space)

Around 2 A.M., there's another energetic shift as we enter a vata time. Insomniacs who have trouble falling asleep will find their eyes open somewhere after this time because of the mind-racing, anxiety-provoking influence of increased vata. These are the hours of our dream state, of the literally rapid movements of REM sleep. Since our intuition, creativity, spiritual connection, and the activity of the nervous system are all governed by vata, this makes sense. If you can't fall back to sleep, try meditating; use the energy around you. If you have a tendency to wake up at this time, your body is saying that you need more restorative, relaxing practices to wind down before bed. These could include nose oil, aromatherapy, yoga poses like legs up against wall, meditation, or ashwagandha (see chapter 10).

SEASONS AS THEY RELATE TO AYURVEDA

Summer

According to Ayurveda, these doshas also cycle through the seasons. Obviously, the summer is the season of the pitta dosha, and our best practices are anything that helps to cool the intensity. Cool sweet fruits, swimming, moonlight walks, mint tea, and coconut water are a few of the remedies that can keep us from overheating and allow us to maintain our YogaLean routines.

Fall/Winter

Fall and early winter is the time or season of vata. This is the time when we may feel darker, dry, empty, anxious, or agitated or have trouble sleeping. Warm comfort foods are the season's remedy. Instead of indulging in pies and cookies in an effort to soothe anxiety, try mashed sweet potatoes, lentil soup, warm drinks, slower yoga practices, meditation in movement, or a massage. Turn up the heat for yoga in a warm room or try sitting in the steam room at the gym or spa.

Winter/Spring

Early winter into spring is the wet, heavy time of kapha as well as the time of new growth. Since this is when we may succumb to seasonal allergies or a flood of mucus, cleansing foods such as dark green leafy vegetables and grains like millet and barley can support our health. This is the time to step up your workout routine and break the most intense sweat of the year—with nature's support.

...

PART TWO

gaining lean consciousness

6

Yoga for a Lean Body

..

"It all starts with the body. The physical is the easiest
and yet most challenging thing to master."

We reach the mind through the body. The more we feel and breathe, the
more likely shifts are to happen.

Gaining Lean Consciousness is putting the lessons into physical
practice through yoga poses and recipes created for a leaner you, high energy,
strengthened immunity, relaxation, and a youthful body. These are the spokes that
you will tangibly put into place in order to shift your lifestyle, the way you feel physically, and the way your body looks through the food you eat and the exercise you do.

Before diving into the YogaLean poses and sequences, I want to go over the importance of technique in order to avoid injury. Every body is unique, as you know, so
it's a matter of properly preparing your body, listening to it, and creating a comfortable environment to succeed in a fluid and safe practice.

Among the many styles of yoga, YogaFit seeks to bring yoga to everybody in
every body. Designed for use in both the fitness and traditional studio environment,
YogaFit vinyasa yoga has the following stylistic elements:

1. **YogaFit Seven Principles of Alignment:** These help us achieve maximum benefit from the poses while reducing the potential for injury.

2. **YogaFit Transformational Language/Inner Dialogue:** These will aid in a key element in maintaining Lean Consciousness, the ability to practice PEP, which is explained on page 81.

3. **YogaFit Three Mountain Format:** This format provides for adequate warmup at the beginning of class, work in the middle section of class, and effective, deep stretching at the end of class.

Safe Yoga differs from traditional yoga in that the postures link in a fluid heat-building way, meaning that the breath is linked with the movements, heating the body naturally and organically.

YogaFit Seven Principles of Alignment

In YogaFit, we express hatha yoga postures using our Seven Principles of Alignment. These principles help to create the optimal biomechanical position for the body during movement and while holding the poses. The Seven Principles of Alignment increase safety while simultaneously providing functional mechanical principles that you can use in your daily life. Remembering these principles of alignment is important in a healthy YogaLean practice and can help to modify the postures and the transitions whenever it is necessary to accommodate your body.

1. **Establishing Base and Dynamic Tension:** Establish a firm base in the feet and hands, stacking your joints for maximum support and contracting your muscles to become stable in a pose.

2. **Creating Core Stability:** Use the muscles of the trunk (for instance, the abdominals and the erector spinae) to create core stability prior to moving into and while holding poses for greater strength and internal support.

3.   **Aligning the Spine:** The spine is supported through core stabilization in all applicable poses, and the head follows the movement of the spine. When moving into twists, flexion, or extension, start in neutral spine.

4.   **Softening and Aligning Knees:** In all applicable poses, the knees stay in line with the ankles and point directly out over the toes. In general, the knees, when bent, will also remain in the same line as the hips. To prevent hyperextension, keep a micro bend in the knees at all times.

5.   **Relaxing Shoulders Back and Down:** The shoulders are drawn naturally back and down in poses to help reduce tension in the neck and shoulders.

6.   **Hinging at the Hips:** When moving into and out of forward bends, hinge from the hips, using the natural pulley system of the ball and socket joint and keeping a micro bend in the knees.

7.   **Shortening the Lever:** When hip hinging, flexing, or extending the spine, keep the arms out to the side or alongside the body to reduce strain on the muscles of the lower back.

Inner Dialogue

Without a positive inner dialogue, you're not going to get very far. Self talk can make or break us. In YogaFit we practice giving PEP (Praise-Encourage-Praise) Feedback to others (for those of you who are hungry, I like to call this a "Slap Sandwich"), and I want you to learn to apply this feedback when communicating with yourself during times of struggle.

In groups, to help each other improve, PEP Feedback is a great way for you to shift your dialogue to carefully support those around you. This format is also used to guide you through self talk and to build a safer inner dialogue when you feel frustrated or need to talk yourself out of something.

Both start with a positive statement, then encourage with a strong help statement, followed by another positive statement. Below are the PEP guidelines when speaking to others. Learning this will help us communicate better in our relationships. Once you gain an understanding of PEP, you can use it on yourself.

Praise ♡ Encourage ♡ Praise

PRINCIPLES OF GIVING CONSTRUCTIVE FEEDBACK

- With an intention of being helpful, supportive, and encouraging, ask permission before providing feedback.
- Focus first on the positive and then on how to improve. Deal only with a specific skill or technique that can be changed.
- Describe the skill or technique rather than evaluating it.
- Relate objectively what specifically was seen or heard. Facts about skill or technique are exact and without exaggeration.
- Use "I" statements to accept responsibility for your own perceptions and emotions.
- Check to make sure that the recipient understood the message in the way it was intended. Avoid making the recipient "wrong" by wanting to be "right."
- Avoid extreme or coercive language like "should," "always," and "never."

PRINCIPLES OF RECEIVING FEEDBACK

- Listen openly, without excuses or judgments of yourself or others.
- When you ask for feedback, be specific in describing the skill or technique about which you want the feedback.
- Let go of defensive reactions or temptations to rationalize the skill or technique at issue.
- Summarize your understanding of the feedback.
- Using "I" statements, share your thoughts and feelings about the feedback.

GUIDELINES FOR EFFECTIVE FEEDBACK EXCHANGE

- Agree to be open and honest with one another. Skills and techniques must be exhibited that demonstrate genuineness. For example, make sure you use nonthreatening body language, tone of voice, and choice of words.
- Take notes! Writing down feedback you receive allows you to refer to it later. This is also a great opportunity to jot down questions about the feedback you are receiving. Listening attentively and questioning for understanding are key to the communication process.
- Phrase comments in positive terms ("I think the Sun Salutation series might be improved by naming each pose").

I practice a lot of self talk. It's so important to be able to talk yourself out a bad situation, whether it's calling an ex or going for that second piece of chocolate cake. Self talk during your yoga practice should be gentle and encouraging; we never want to curse our hamstrings for being tight. Learn to watch your inner dialogue, and learn how you respond to your own inner coach best. Your inner coach needs to have a few voices and tones.

For example, if I am talking to myself about eating on a more regular basis, which is an issue I have, I may say in PEP:

P: Beth, you are doing a great job with your commitment to your health.

E: Perhaps it would be helpful for you to remember to eat every three to four hours so that you can keep your blood sugar levels even and keep your energy up.

P: Know that you can refine your commitment to your health.

You must learn to be firm but gentle with yourself. Your boot camp coach needs to be able to get you to the gym every day and make you work hard. Your inner therapist coach needs to be able to tell you it's okay if you have eaten two pizzas and not beat you up—as well as to help you understand your behaviors. The best inner coach you can develop is one that consistently moves you toward greatness. With time, practice, and witness consciousness, you will be able to shift your inner dialogue to work *for* you and not against you.

Your inner coach should be your best advocate always and help you achieve your goals.

Three Mountain Format

*I work in the Three Mountain Format, which is warmup, work, and cool down, with sug-*gested modifications and options on most poses. During your pose sequences, I encourage you to apply the essence of YogaFit—listening to your body; letting go of judgment, expectation, and competition; being present in the moment and in your practice—to keep your body safe. If you tap into your mind, you will be immersed in a transformative experience.

In YogaFit, we apply modern exercise science to the ancient mind/body practice of yoga. While yoga can have a profound impact on the physical, emotional, and spiritual health of students, improper sequencing and pacing create opportunities for physical discomfort and injury. For this reason, I ask you to use the following format to establish full readiness and benefits from your poses.

- Mountain 1:   Warmup phase
- Mountain 2:   Work phase
- Mountain 3:   Cool-down phase

In addition to these three phases, you will use two "valleys," which are extensions of Mountain 1 and Mountain 2, respectively:

- Valley 1:   Sun salutations
- Valley 2:   Upright standing balance poses

Importance of Warmup and Cool Down

Warming up the body completely with large body moves prior to engaging in any complex or flexibility-oriented pose is important to prep the muscles, especially if your workout environment is cold. Many assume that stretching prior to exercise or an athletic event helps to prepare the muscles for the activity and reduce injury. However, the scientific literature has not, to date, confirmed that flexibility exercises, performed before elevation of core body temperature, are effective in reducing injury. Since yoga is a form of exercise that requires a combination of flexibility, strength, endurance, and coordination, I want you to stretch at the end.

The human body is composed of a number of structures: skeletal, muscular, nervous, circulatory, and so on. The muscular structure of the body provides movement and protection for the skeletal system. All actions in the body take place through the contraction or relaxation of muscles at the major joints of the body. Each of these joints has an inherent range of motion due to the configuration of the bones in the body. However, this range of motion can be restricted by the ability of the soft tissues of the body, including the muscles, tendons (which attach muscle to bones), and ligaments (which connect bones), to accommodate the range. Muscles can become tense due to many factors, including stress and working joints through a restricted range of motion. The result is perceived inflexibility.

The solution to increasing flexibility is to begin working the joints through the full range of motion, which "stretches" the muscles and, to a lesser degree, the tendons. Two essential properties of muscles allow them to stretch: elasticity and plasticity. The elastic properties of muscles allow them to return back to their original state from a stretch. If this were not the case, muscles would lengthen continuously until they had become so loose that no movement would be possible! The plastic properties of muscles allow them to adapt to the continued stresses that we place on them and retain these adaptations. If muscles were not plastic, then we would not be able to strengthen or stretch them; they would just stay the same after each activity. Interestingly, both of these qualities become more evident when there is an elevation in core body temperature. Another way of saying this is that muscles respond better if we work them when they are warm.

Therefore, the most appropriate place to introduce deep stretching (and even strength and endurance work) is after an elevation in body temperature sufficient to increase the potential for elasticity and plasticity in our muscles. Consequently, all physical exercise, including yoga, should begin with warmups that elevate core body temperature and use the full range of motion in the major joints. Once we have sufficiently elevated the core body temperature, we can then begin using movements that condition the body for greater strength, stretch, and flexibility. Our deepest flexibility stretches should occur near the end of class, when the body is warmest and elasticity and plasticity in the muscles are optimal.

Before applying this to your yoga practice, know that fitness moves are incorporated, such as sit-ups and push-ups, lunge and hold. Transitions are smooth from pose to pose with the focus on a full-body workout; all body parts are worked equally. Modifications and levels are offered to suit the needs of several different students at different levels in the room. Encourage yourself to take breaks; *let go* of expectations, judgment, and competition; and do not push yourself past your limits—you will know when you've reached your limit if you listen and feel the signs your body is giving you.

WARMUP SEQUENCE

Flight of the Bird (5 to 7 minutes, one breath for each movement; see page 94)

Chair Flow (5 times; see page 106)

Sun Salutation (7 on each side; see page 87)

Flow Series (7 times; see page 98)

Cat and Cow (10 to 15 times, one breath for each movement; see page 96)

COOLDOWN SEQUENCE (HOLD EACH POSE FOR TEN DEEP BREATHS)

Lying Down Spinal Twist (see page 132)

Bridge (see page 128)

Upside Down Pigeon (see page 134)

Reclining Butterfly (see page 136)

Dead Bug (see page 138)

Energy

Energy will get us through the day, will make us laugh, give us the ability to cook at home, or incorporate a more active lifestyle. The combination of these poses will stimulate our body and target our muscles and limbs specifically for increased energy and metabolism.

1. Sun Salutation
2. Sunflower
3. Flight of the Bird
4. Cat and Cow
5. Flow Series
6. Camel

Sun Salutation

GETTING INTO THE POSE

Begin in Mountain pose: standing straight, feet shoulder-width apart, shoulders relaxed, and head in line with the spine. From Mountain, inhale, sweeping your arms up (A). Exhaling, bend your knees and Swan Dive into Forward Fold (B). Inhaling, step your right foot back into a Lunge, left knee over ankle (C). Exhaling, step your left foot back into Downward Facing Dog. Inhale into Plank (D), keeping your core strong and your back straight.

Shift forward onto your toes, exhale into Crocodile, lowering your shoulders to align with your elbows, hips, and heels (E). Inhaling, pulling forward from the core, come on to the tops of your feet for Upward Facing Dog (F, G). Exhale into Downward Facing Dog (H). Inhaling, step your right foot forward into Lunge. Exhaling, step your left foot forward into Forward Fold. Inhaling and bending your knees, circle-sweep your arms up into Mountain. Exhaling, sit back into Chair.

Repeat the sequence on the other side by extending your legs and sweeping your arms up to come into Mountain with arms raised. (Then start again at the second step of this sequence.)

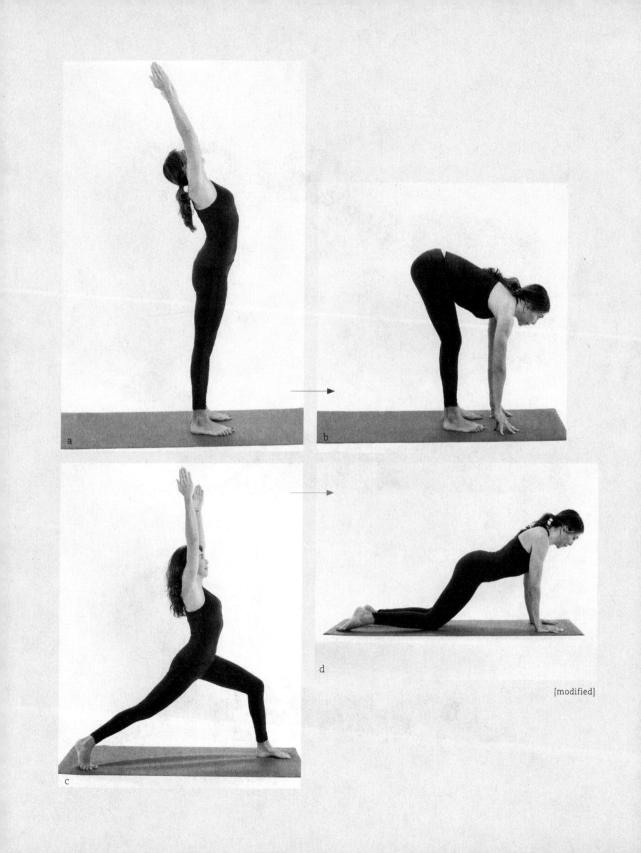

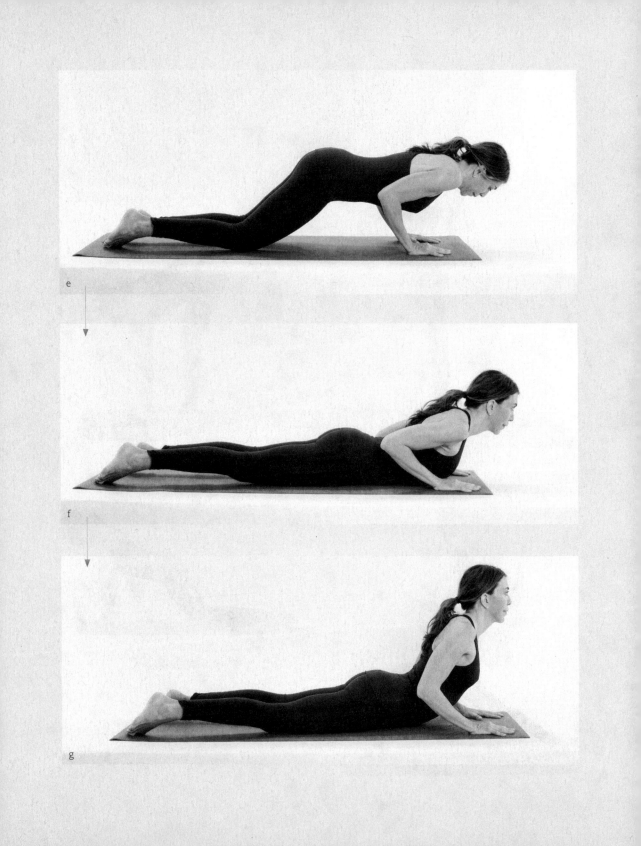

e

f

g

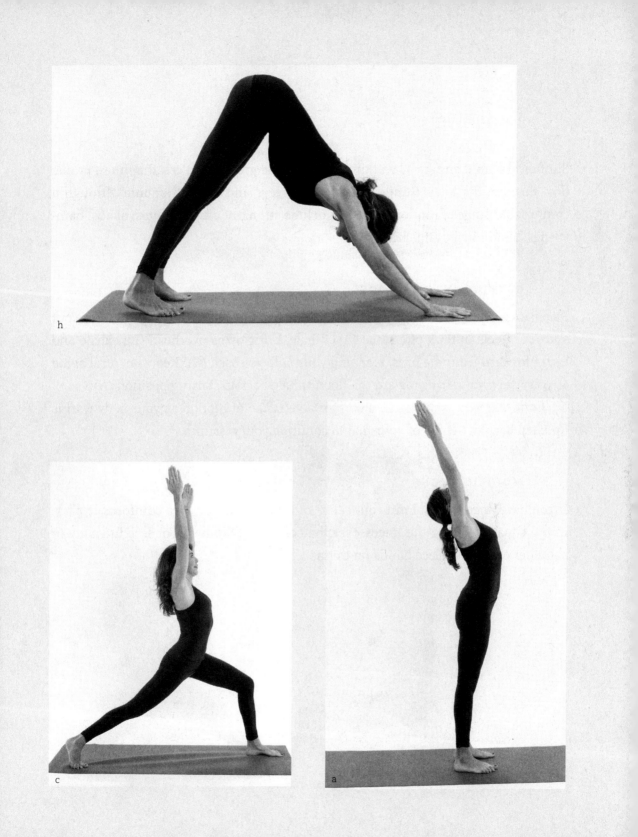

Sunflower

Sunflowers build energy by working large muscle groups and creating more pranic flow through the body. Sunflowers work the legs and move the joints through a comfortable range of motion. Benefits include strengthening of glutes, quads, hamstrings, abdominals, and shoulders.

GETTING INTO THE POSE

Step back to face the long edge of your mat. Open your thighs and turn your toes out and your heels in for a plié squat (A). Inhale, bring arms overhead (B); exhale and hinge forward from the hips, reaching your tailbone back (C). Keep a neutral spine as you sweep your arms toward the floor. Inhale back to starting position (A).

Continue to move through a comfortable range of motion as your body warms up. Step back to the top of your mat to continue your warmup.

MODIFICATIONS

If you have knee issues, limit your range of motion and stay in a comfortable place in the squat, pointing the knees over the centers of the feet. For less intensity or shoulder concerns, place hands on thighs.

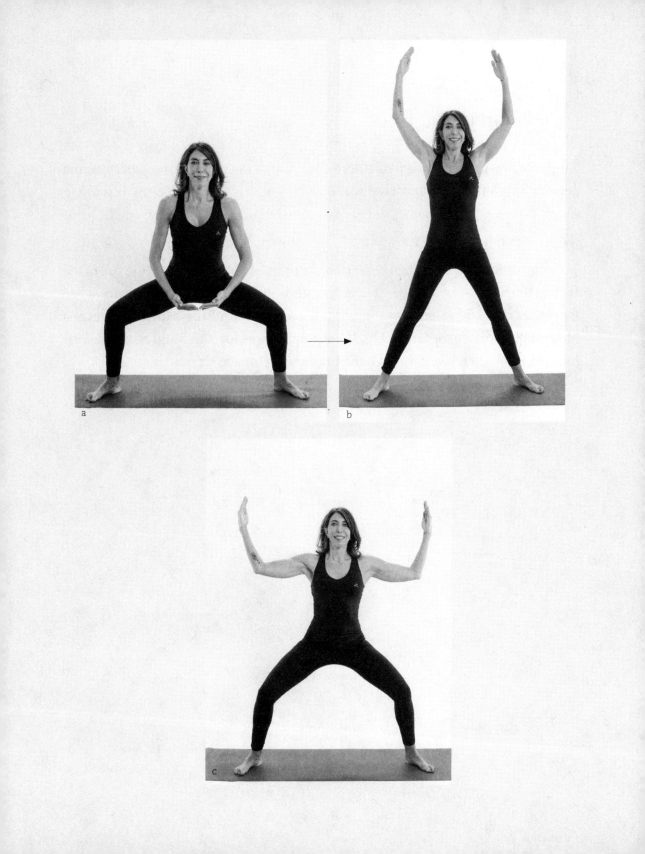

a

b

c

Flight of the Bird

Targets the respiratory and circulatory systems, creating a lot of internal space, and gets you into a flow state quickly and easily.

GETTING INTO THE POSE

Start out standing in Mountain pose; step the right foot back and plant the ball of the foot on the floor—like a lunge—but keep your front foot flat. Extend your arms like the wings of a bird. Step forward, wrap the arms around the body like a hug in Mountain pose, step the left foot back, extend the arms like the wings of a bird. Step forward and keep flowing through the movements for 3 to 5 minutes.

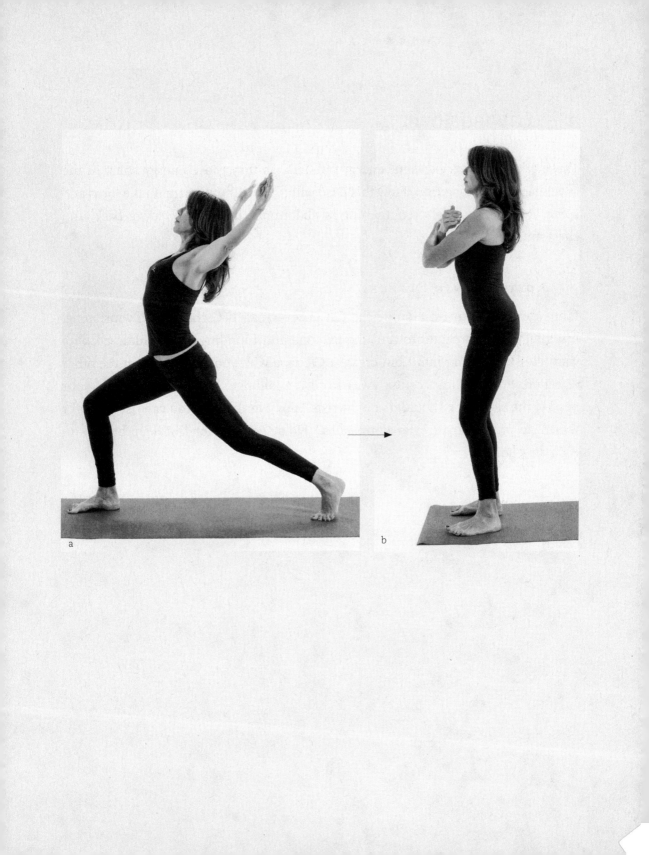

Cat and Cow

These two poses are excellent energy builders, as they move energy stuck in the lower back and midsection. Flow this pose with the breath to warm up the torso and spine. Benefits include strengthening of abdominal, upper back, lower back, and chest muscles.

GETTING INTO THE POSE

From hands and knees, assume the Cat pose—create a C shape with your spine, bringing the heart center toward the tailbone and rounding your middle back toward the sky. Moving into Cow, create a C shape with your spine, but in the other direction. Pull the heart center away from the tailbone, lifting the crown of your head to the sky. Stack shoulders over wrists, hips over knees. (You can use "fists for wrists" to prevent hyperextension issues.) Hold the pose for five deep breaths in each direction.

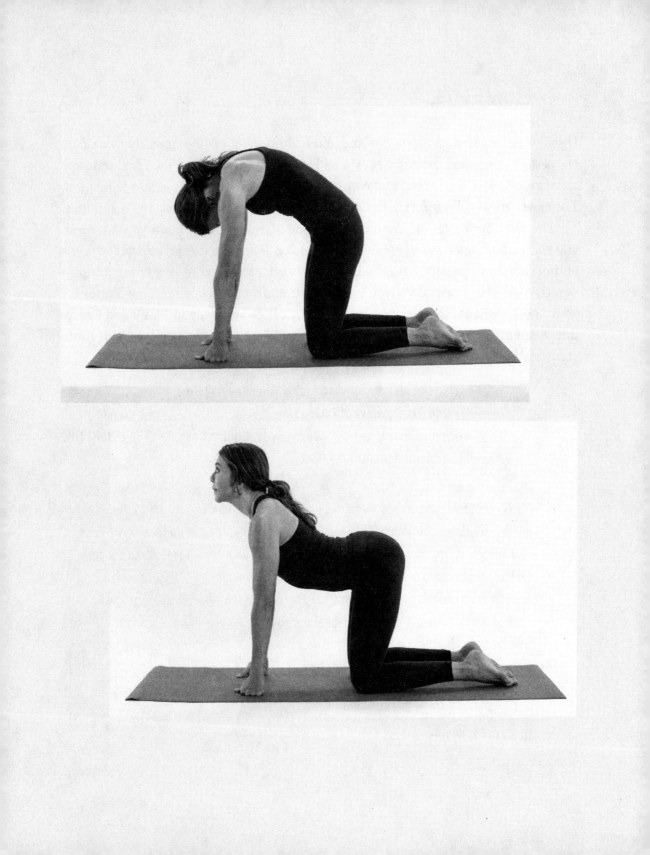

Flow Series

If you were stranded on a desert island and had no weight equipment, this would be the perfect upper body strengthener. The Flow Series, also called the Half Series, is a dynamic flow of four poses that constitute the "bottom" half of the Sun Salutation. The Flow Series builds upper body and core strength while also increasing endurance.

The Flow Series can be done on or off the knees, depending on your strength and ability. Both options target the same muscles. While this series appears to focus entirely on the upper body, it actually depends on a strong core. If you are a beginner, start on your knees until you have the strength to practice the Flow Series off your knees without struggling or dropping your hips and belly in Plank and Crocodile. Remember to keep your hands shoulder-width apart or closer if that feels more comfortable for your body.

FLOW SERIES: Downward Facing Dog (see page 91), Plank, Upward Facing Dog (D), Downward Facing Dog

MODIFIED FLOW SERIES (KNEELING): Child's Pose, Kneeling Plank (B), Kneeling Crocodile (A), Child's Pose

Plank and Child's Pose are two starting positions you will use in the Flow Series. Plank strengthens abdominals, lower back, chest, shoulders, and triceps, while Child's Pose strengthens the mind-body connection and stretches the lower back, glutes, and shoulders.

Plank is entered from Downward-Facing Dog. Shift forward until your shoulders are directly above your wrists. Press your heels back toward the wall behind you. Reach forward through the crown of your head. Keep your back straight and your abdominals firm.

For Child's Pose, begin kneeling on all fours. Push back and bring your arms around to the side of your body. Rest and breathe, allowing your body to completely relax.

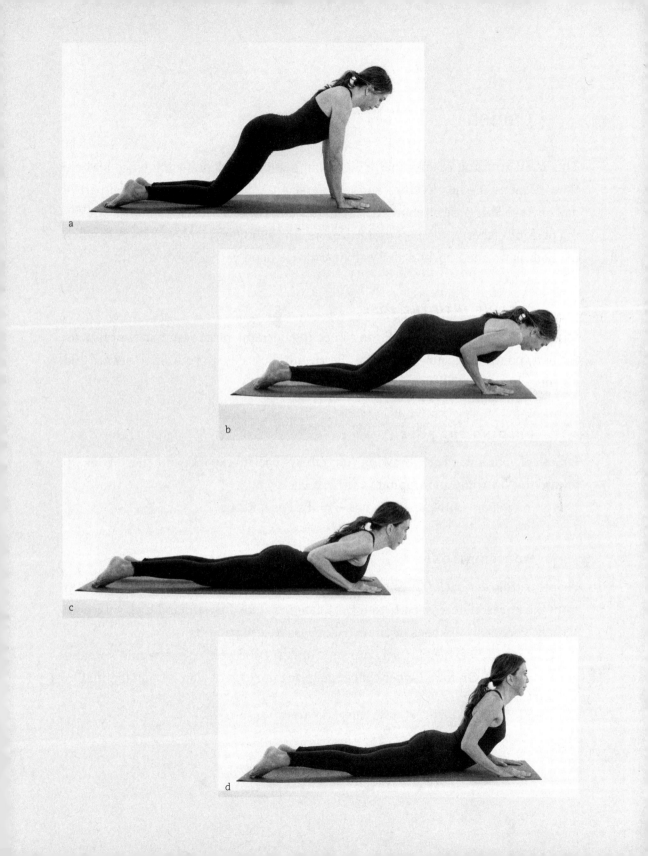

Camel

This is an amazing opener that is energizing and creates self-confidence and chi flow. It opens the heart center and counteracts the forward flexion that is part of daily living. This pose strengthens the glutes and the lower back as well as stretching pectorals (chest), intercostals, hip flexors, and shoulders. Only do this pose when the body is warmed up, and always follow a back bend with a forward bend.

GETTING INTO THE POSE

Move slowly, feeling your way. From a kneeling position, place your hands or fists on the bony points alongside your spine. Firm your glutes. Push your hips forward and lift your chest to the sky.

HOLDING THE POSE

Lift out of your lower back, drawing your elbows back to expand your chest. Look up toward the sky without dropping your head back.

As you get out of the pose, go into Child's Pose. Rest.

MODIFICATIONS

People with lower back issues or injuries should be cautious. Use chest expansion from the knees, if necessary. If your neck fatigues, look forward and tuck your chin slightly. For sensitive knees or another knee issue, use padding.

Take it to the next level: Curl your toes under. Drop your arms behind you and grab your heels. Or, for a bigger challenge, place the tops of your feet on the mat.

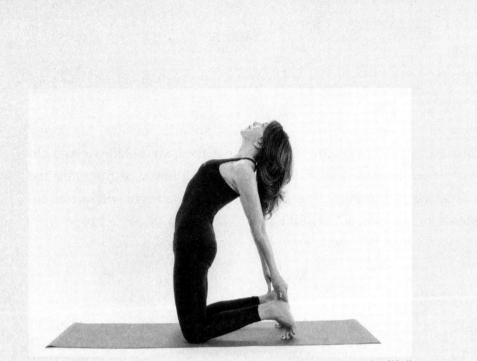

[modified]

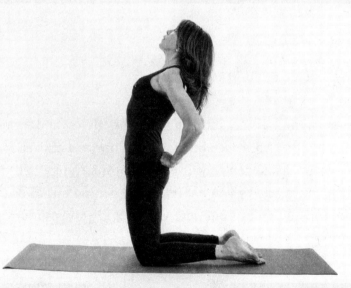

[modified]

Lean

Aside from gaining an overall Lean Consciousness, specific practices can trigger your body for a leaner you. The core is the nucleus of the body, holding it together to help you stand upright, move gracefully, and function. Without a strong core, the rest of your body will feel negative effects, which is why we begin with a core sequence that leads into the rest of the workout.

1. Core Work
2. Boat
3. Chair Flow
4. Twisting Chair
5. Warrior I
6. Warrior II
7. Triangle

Core Work

A strong midsection, including the abs, glutes, and lower back muscles, assists us in everything from deep breathing to improved efficiency and athletic performance. A strong, stable center will increase your energy and quite literally support just about every activity you do, including getting out of bed in the morning. Furthermore, conditioning your core will go a long way toward preventing back pain and injury.

Working your core will do far more for you than build strong muscles. When your core is strong, you feel strong. In other words, abdominal exercises will strengthen your power center (midsection), enhancing your self-esteem and boosting positive energy. Practicing them regularly will help you listen to your gut and use your gut to release serotonin (a relaxer) and trust what you know. A powerful midsection will enhance the qualities of your third chakra, strengthening your will-power, personal power, determination, and discipline. (See appendix A.)

Step One: On your back, lie down with knees bent. Interlace your hands behind your head. Engage your glutes and press your lower back against the floor. Lift your back ribs off the floor, squeeze at the top and release—repeat 20 to 30 times.

Step Two: Raise your feet off the floor; go elbow to opposite knee, add a center lift, and raise your tailbone off the floor for more work.

Step Three: Extend your legs to the sky—reach your hands up and touch your feet. Repeat 10 to 20 times—if your neck gets tired, support it with your hands.

Step Four: Bicycle your legs, taking elbow to opposite knee. Repeat 20 to 30 times.

Step Five: From a seated position, place your legs in front of you with your knees bent. Grab the backs of your legs and sit upright, keeping your spine extended. Lean back till you feel resistance in your abs and then lift one inch; hold and then pull forward. Work within your own range of motion, moving forward and back. Do 3 sets of 20. Finish with Knees to Chest pose (see p. 122).

Boat

Boat pose is an amazing core strengthener, because it activates your power center. Boat pose strengthens the abdominals, hip flexors, and quadriceps as well as targets the back muscles. The pose strengthens the core and improves balance.

GETTING INTO THE POSE

Sitting upright on the floor, bend your knees and hold on to your hamstrings. Slowly lift one foot at a time away from the floor, keeping your back straight. Reach forward with your arms as you balance on the backs of your glutes.

HOLDING THE POSE

Focus on your breath to lengthen your spine and lift your chest, relaxing your shoulders backward and down.

Take it to the next level: Straighten your legs and reach forward without rounding your back.

MODIFICATIONS

If you have back injuries or are a beginner, keep your feet on the floor and continue holding your hamstrings.

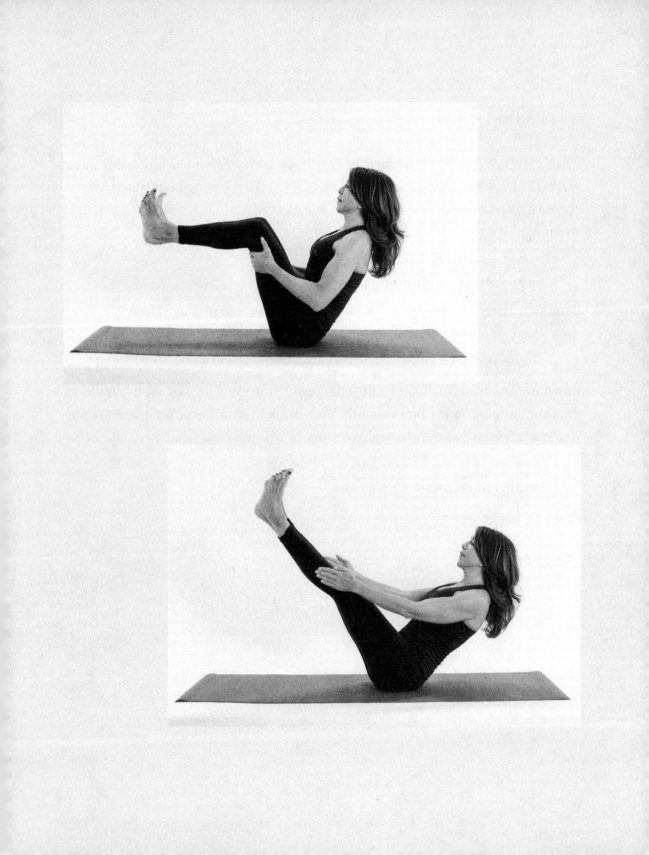

Chair Flow

Chair Flow is a great workout for the lower body. It creates a lot of heat quickly as it works the largest muscle groups in the body. Chair Flow strengthens quads, glutes, shoulders, and core. To flow we move in and out of Chair Flow with every breath to warm up.

GETTING INTO THE POSE

Bend your knees and drop your buttocks, as if you were sitting in a chair.

HOLDING THE POSE

Reach back with your tailbone. Lift your chest to the sky. Lift your arms parallel to the floor, keeping your elbows slightly bent. Support your lower back by engaging your core. Keep your knees behind your toes by shifting your weight to your heels.

MODIFICATIONS

Rest your hands on your thighs for more support.

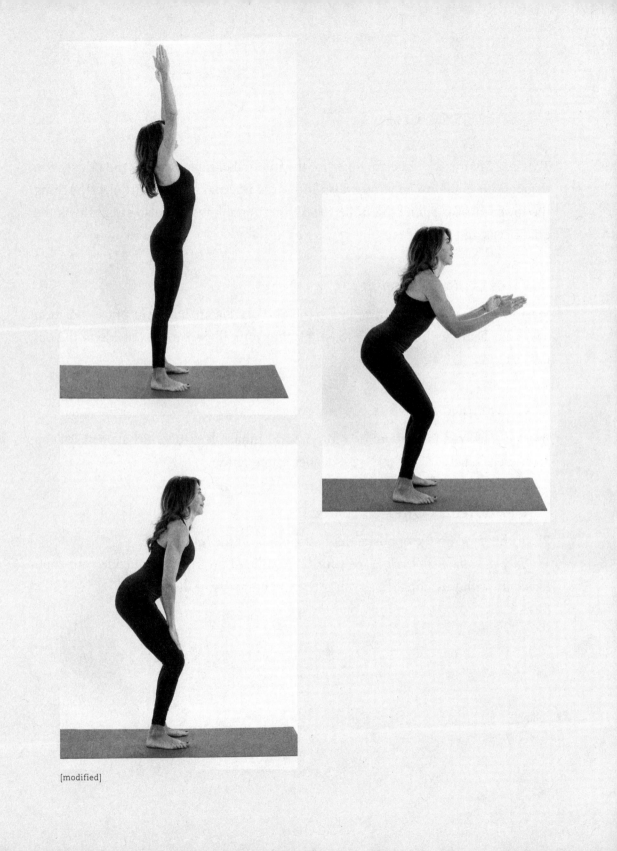

[modified]

Twisting Chair

Twisting Chair is a wonderful toner for the internal organs and puts the midsection through the motions. This pose also improves internal organ function, stretching the lower lumbar spine, the upper back, and the obliques. It also strengthens the quadriceps and the glutes.

GETTING INTO THE POSE

Start in Chair pose. Lengthen your spine and place your hands in prayer position over your heart. Twist from the waist, placing your elbow on the outside of the opposite thigh.

HOLDING THE POSE

Engage your core to support your lower back. Inhale, lengthen. Exhale, twist. Keep your knees together as you release deeper into rotation.

MODIFICATIONS

Place one hand on the opposite thigh, the other on the lower back.

Take it to the next level: Place your bottom hand on the floor outside your foot. Reach up with your top arm as you roll your chest toward the sky.

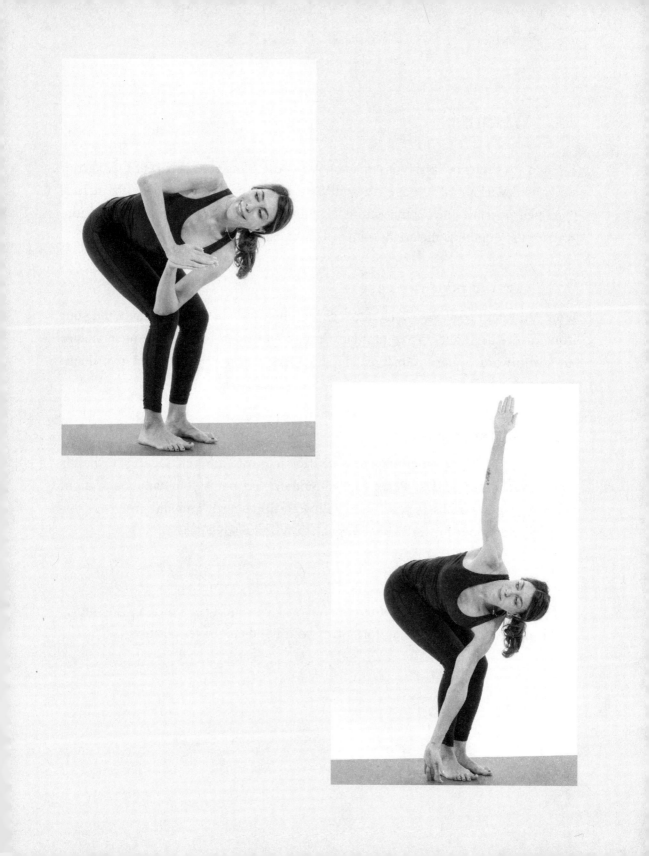

Warrior I

Tap into your warrior spirit with this powerful pose. This pose is part of the Warrior series (see Warrior II on page 112 and Warrior III on page 148). Benefits include increased physical and mental strength, and enhanced power and determination. Warrior I strengthens the quads, glutes, lats, upper back, and shoulders.

GETTING INTO THE POSE

From Mountain pose, step back into a short lunge and align your heels. Bend your front knee, stacking it over your ankle. Straighten your back leg, turning your toes slightly forward. Square your hips and shoulders with the front of your mat. Raise your arms to the sky.

HOLDING THE POSE

Continue to press the outer edge of your back foot into the mat. Open your hands and activate your fingers. Relax your shoulders and point your tailbone straight down. Engage your abs as you lift up with your upper body and sink into your forward leg. Keep your forward knee over your ankle. Switch sides.

MODIFICATIONS

To decrease the intensity, straighten the forward leg slightly or shorten your stance. In the event of shoulder discomfort, bring your hands to prayer position.

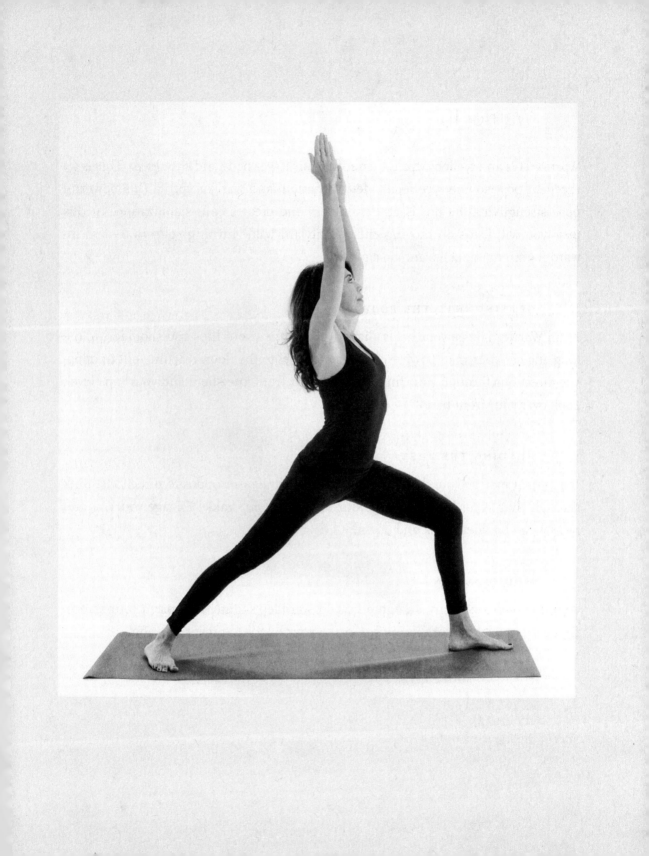

Warrior II

Warrior II is an excellent strengthener for your lower body and shoulders. This is an excellent pose to enhance focus, determination, and warrior spirit. This powerful pose strengthens the quads and shoulders and creates core stabilization. In this pose you will focus on moving energy outward while turning your awareness inward for strength, focus, and discipline.

GETTING INTO THE POSE

From Warrior I, keep your heels aligned as you open your hips and shoulders to the long edge of your mat. Lower your arms parallel to the floor, reaching out in opposite directions through your fingers. Keep your front knee bent and your hips level. Look over your front hand.

HOLDING THE POSE

Lift your upper body and reach through your fingers in opposite directions. Sink through your lower body, keeping your knee over your ankle. Engage your abs and relax your shoulders back and down.

MODIFICATIONS

To decrease the intensity, straighten the forward leg slightly or shorten your stance. In the event of shoulder discomfort, bring your hands to prayer position.

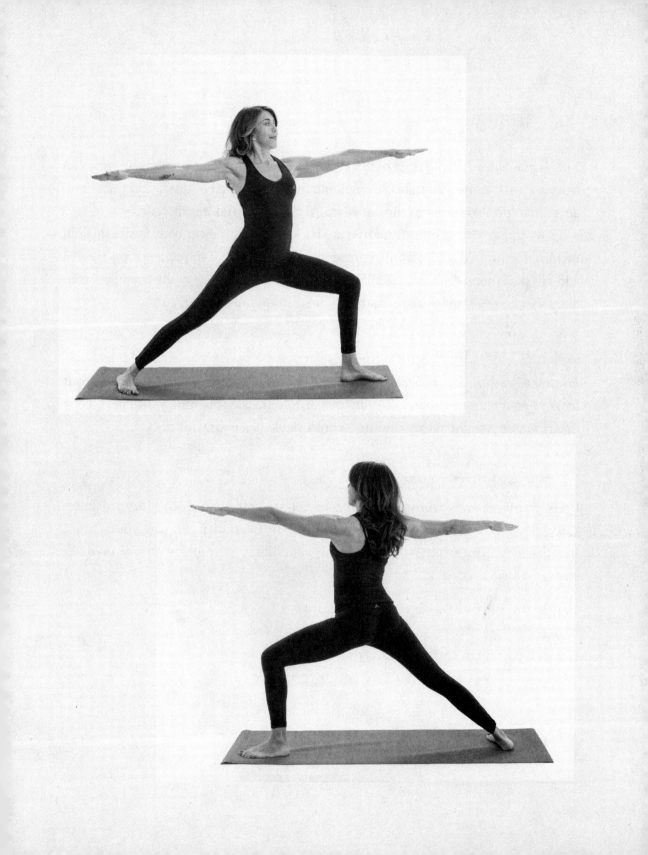

Triangle

This is one of my favorite yoga poses. It moves energy in four directions, originating from a strong center. Triangle strengthens the quads, the obliques, and the shoulders. Triangle also stretches the hamstrings, pectorals, and intercostals.

Your upper body is lifting and moving back while your lower body is sinking and moving forward. Triangle pose represents creating for ourselves a strong mental and physical foundation, represented by the two bottom points of the triangle. From here, we can begin to look up, exploring the third point—the spiritual.

GETTING INTO THE POSE

From the Warrior II pose, straighten your front leg. Reach forward, then lower your hand to your shin or ankle. Lift your back arm to the sky, opening your chest. Look up, down, or straight ahead, finding a comfortable place for your neck.

HOLDING THE POSE

Press your feet away from each other, keeping a soft bend in the forward knee. Check that your nose stays over your leg, not in front of it. Engage your glutes. Breathe length into your spine, allowing your inner strength to fuel your outer strength. Switch sides.

MODIFICATIONS

If your hamstrings are tight, place your lower hand on a block.

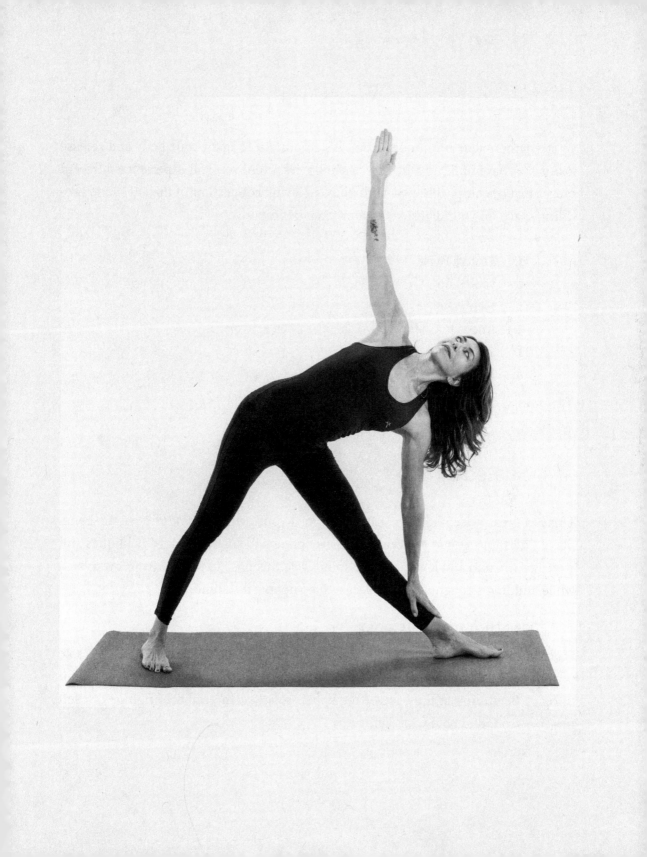

Immunity

To strengthen your immune system, it's important to open your body and release toxins that have built up and may cause illness. Here you will experience different moves that open up your chest and body, relieving congestion in the chest and providing space for your digestive system to work properly.

1. Seated Twist
2. Table Top
3. Fish Pose
4. Knees to Chest
5. Twisting Lunge
6. Lateral Flexion
7. Bridge

Seated Twist

This is a great twist where you can really go at your own pace and receive the benefits of a twist in a gentle way. This pose strengthens the upper back and obliques and stretches the mid and lower lumbar spine. Use this pose to release your lower back while building strength in the muscles that support the spine.

GETTING INTO THE POSE

From a seated position, extend your legs out. Bring your right knee up with the sole of your foot on the floor. Place your right hand next to you or behind you and sit upright. Beginning at the base of the spine, rotate to the right, bringing your left forearm around to hold your right shin.

HOLDING THE POSE

Use core strength against your arm to deepen the twist. Lengthen your spine with every inhale; twist further with every exhale. Switch sides.

MODIFICATIONS

If your lower back rounds, sit on a rolled-up yoga mat or folded blanket.

Take it to the next level: Use core strength against your arm to deepen the twist. Place your left elbow outside your right knee. Hold and breathe.

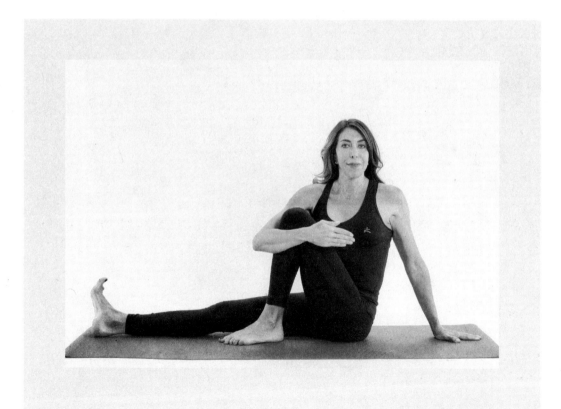

Table Top

This simple pose will stretch out your shoulders, chest, abs, and spine.

GETTING INTO THE POSE

From a seated position, place your hands on the floor behind your body with fists into floor or fingertips facing hips. Place your feet under your knees. Press up like a table top.

HOLDING THE POSE

Engage your glutes and triceps and don't let your table sag. Hold for 10 to 20 deep breaths.

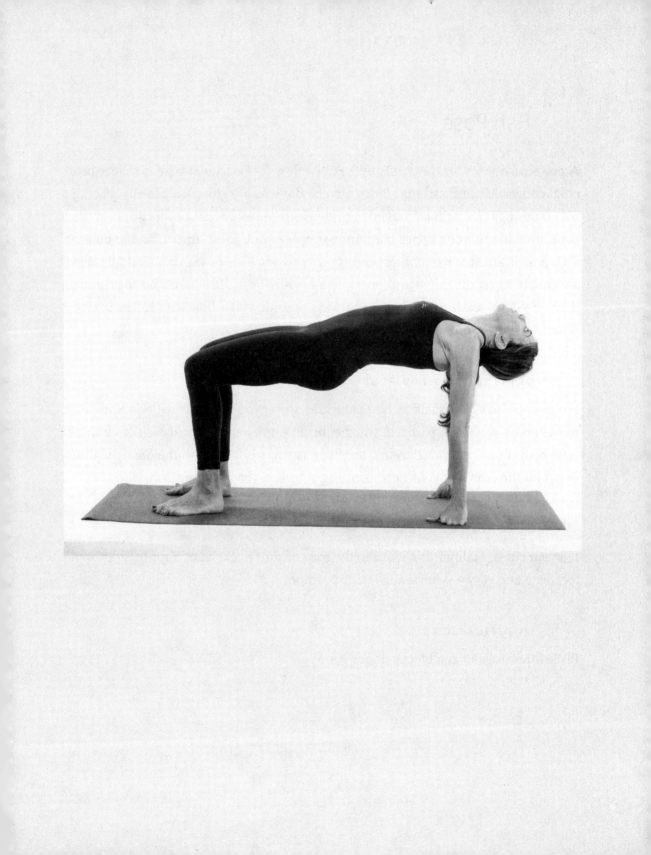

Fish Pose

A powerful opener for the chest and heart center. This is a great pose to relieve bronchial congestion and asthma. It can also be done as a restorative pose by placing a rolled-up yoga mat or folded blanket under your upper back for more support. Fish pose strengthens your upper back and stretches your chest, throat, and shoulders. Fish pose is an effective counter-pose for inversions. This pose can potentially alleviate certain chest disorders and promote a healthy heart. It is also said to stimulate the thyroid, increasing metabolism. Always precede and follow with Knees to Chest pose to stabilize your spine and the muscles in your back.

GETTING INTO THE POSE

From Knees to Chest position (see page 122), lower your legs to the floor. Slide your hands under your hips, palms down, and bring your elbows toward each other under your body. Point your toes toward the floor as you reach back in the opposite direction with the crown of your head, shifting your body back slightly as well.

HOLDING THE POSE

Lift your chest. Maintaining space in the back of your neck, relax. Your breath should feel deep and easy—if not, adjust your position.

MODIFICATIONS

Place three YogaFit egg blocks under your back.

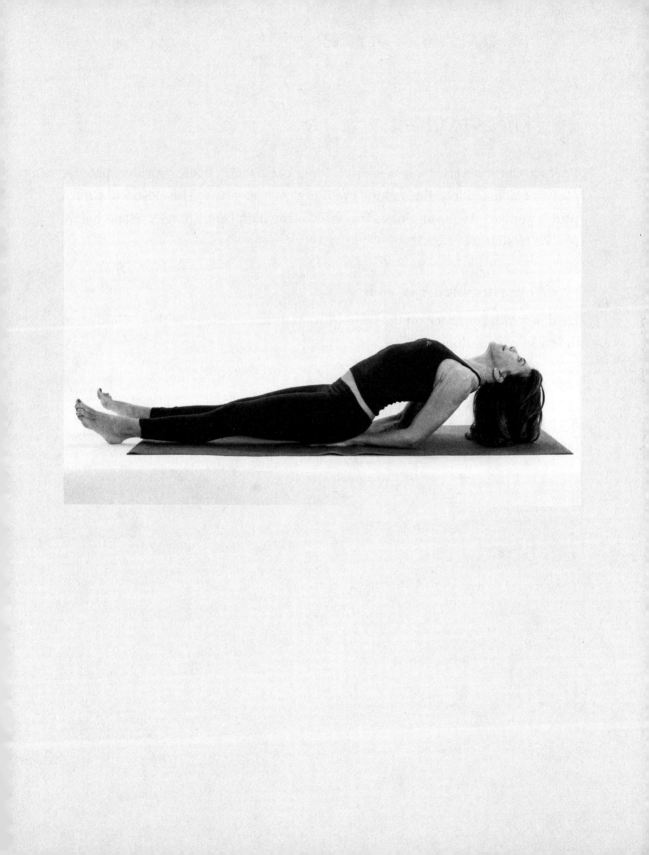

Knees to Chest

Knees to Chest is a great way to alleviate lower back issues. It also provides space for your stomach and intestines in the event of digestive issues. This pose will stretch your lower back and your glutes. Use it following back bends to release and relieve tension in your lower back.

GETTING INTO THE POSE

Lie down with your back on the floor. Bring your knees into your chest. Hold on to the backs of your thighs.

HOLDING THE POSE

Keep drawing your knees toward your chest while keeping your tailbone on the floor. For a gentle back massage, rock side to side.

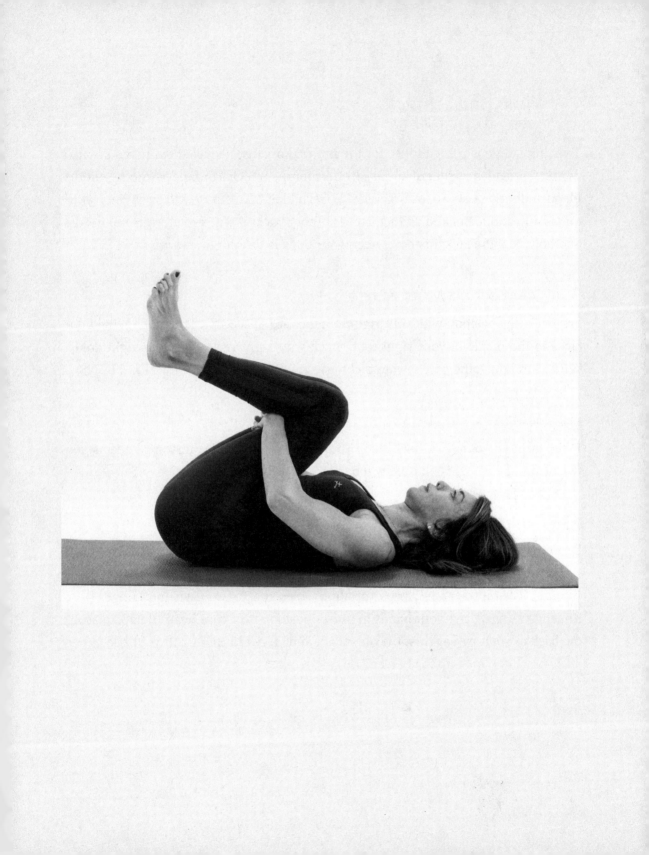

Twisting Lunge

Twisting Lunge is a great toner for the internal organs; like all standing and seated twists, it provides a squeeze-and-soak effect for the internal organs, wringing out the blood and then flushing the organs with fresh blood. This pose will strengthen your quads, hip adductors and abductors, and upper back. It will stretch your hip flexors and obliques. Practice this pose when your body is thoroughly warm.

GETTING INTO THE POSE

From a lunge position with your right foot forward, place your left hand on the floor close to the inside of your right foot. Stack your right knee over your right ankle. With a straight spine, sweep your right arm up, reaching toward the sky.

HOLDING THE POSE

Press through your back heel. Keep your chest close to your forward knee as you twist from the waist. Look up. Switch sides.

MODIFICATIONS

Drop your back knee to the mat for a Kneeling Lunge.

Place your bottom hand on a block to help lengthen the spine for rotation.

Take it to the next level: Try a variation called the Prayer Twisting Lunge: Do a Kneeling Lunge, place your hands in prayer position over your heart. Rotate, placing the back of your arm against the outside of your forward thigh. Lift your back knee off the mat and look up for Prayer Twisting Lunge.

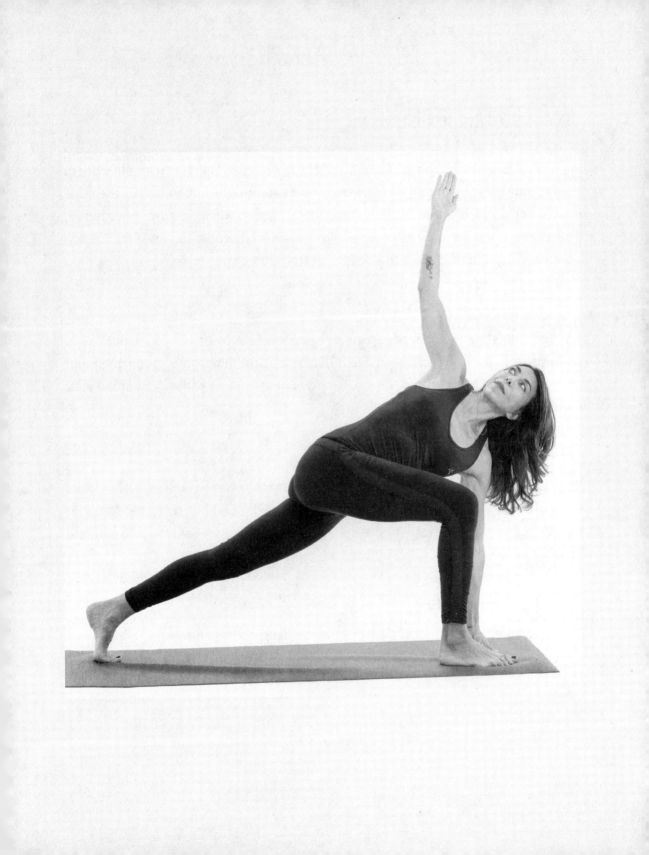

Lateral Flexion

A great pose for the lymphatic system and the lymph glands that run up the sides of the body under the armpits. This pose provides an opportunity to stretch the sides of your body, which you rarely get to do. Lateral Flexion will strengthen your quads, glutes, and intercostals. This pose will stretch your lats and obliques. Practice this pose between standing poses to stretch and strengthen your torso.

GETTING INTO THE POSE

Lift both arms over your head. Create dynamic tension by lifting your upper body and pressing down through your feet. Slide one hand down your outer thigh and reach your other hand toward the sky. Gently lean to the side without dropping your chest.

HOLDING THE POSE

Keep your glutes engaged to protect and support your lower back; breathe into your sides, rib cage, waist, and chest. Keep your head in line with your spine. Don't let your upper body fall forward. Come up and switch sides. Move side to side with the breath.

MODIFICATIONS

For more lower back support, place your lower hand on your hip.

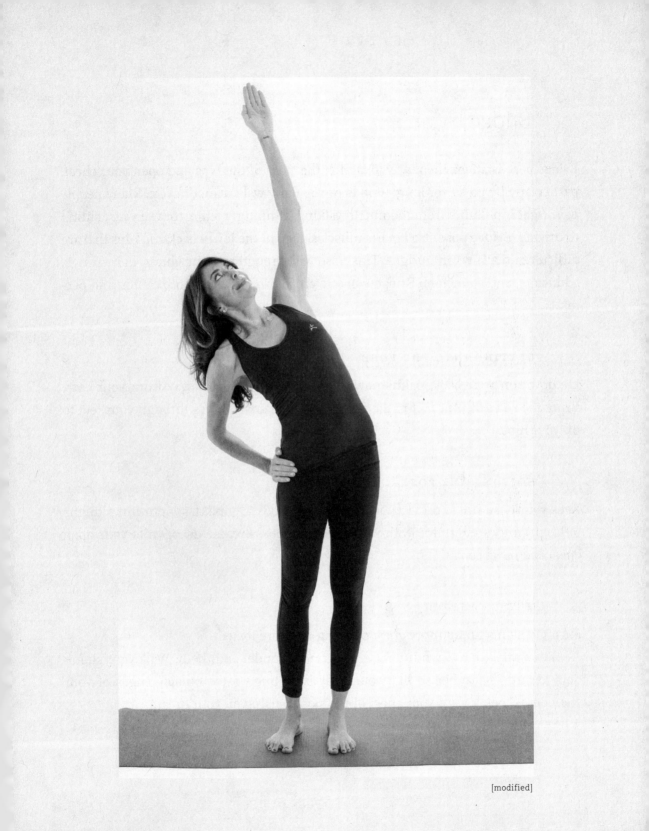

[modified]

Bridge

Bridge pose is an excellent way to stretch the front of the hips and open your chest, particularly if you sit for long periods or regularly walk, run, or cycle. Many people have tight hip flexors from too much walking, running, cycling, or even just sitting or driving. Bridge pose also targets muscles deep in the lower back and hips that are difficult to reach when upright. This pose will strengthen your glutes, hamstrings, adductors, and abductors. Bridge will stretch your hip flexors, core center, and pectorals.

GETTING INTO THE POSE

Lie down on your back, palms down. Slide your shoulders away from your ears. Bring the soles of your feet to the floor, hip-width apart. Press through your feet to lift your hips.

HOLDING THE POSE

Keep your head still to protect your neck—don't look around. Use your inner thighs to keep your knees in line with your hips and toes. Breathe deeply into your open chest and navel center.

MODIFICATIONS

Turn the palms up for more chest opening and core focus.

Take it to the next level: Interlace your fingers under your body. Walk your shoulders toward each other so that your body is resting on the outside edges of your shoulders. Look toward your chest or the sky, focusing on your breath.

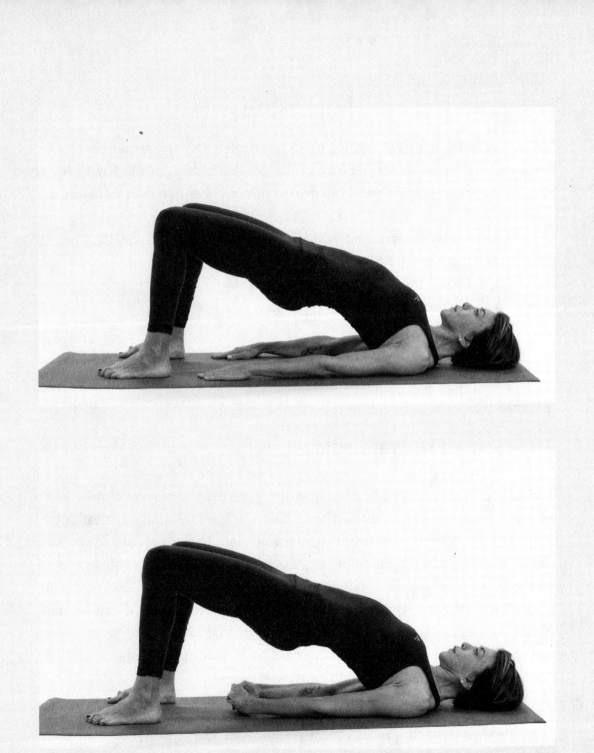

[modified]

Relaxation

Before a long day or after a long day, these poses will help you lengthen your limbs, focus on breathing, and get you into a mind-set that puts your mind and body at ease. This routine will give you a moment to reflect, check into internal being, and reset yourself.

1. Seated Forward Fold
2. Lying Down Spinal Twist
3. Upside Down Pigeon
4. Reclining Butterfly
5. Dead Bug
6. Final Relaxation
7. Legs Up Against Wall

Seated Forward Fold

Forward Folds are cooling and relaxing poses. More than 80 percent of Americans experience some lower back discomfort in their lifetimes. Holding and breathing in Forward Folds will not only help lengthen your tight hamstrings and lower back muscles, it will also relax you, combating the harmful effects of stress on your mind and body. Anytime you are holding a forward bend or when your head is moving toward the earth (as in Downward Dog), practice a sinking breath. Focus on completing your exhale and elongating and releasing muscles from the backs of your legs, up your spine, perhaps even to that tight place between your ears.

GETTING INTO THE POSE

From a seated position, extend your legs. Pull your toes back toward your body. Reach forward, placing your hands on your legs, ankles, or feet or the floor. Using your abs, draw forward through the top of your head.

HOLDING THE POSE

Using a sinking breath, continue to lengthen through your heart and head. Firm your quads. Relax your shoulders back and down. Enjoy the stretch.

MODIFICATIONS

For tight hamstrings, sit on a folded blanket or a rolled-up yoga mat, use a strap or towel around your feet, or bend your knees.

Take it to the next level: Bend one knee, bringing your foot flat to the floor, toes pointing forward. Keeping your knee pointing straight up, reach forward.

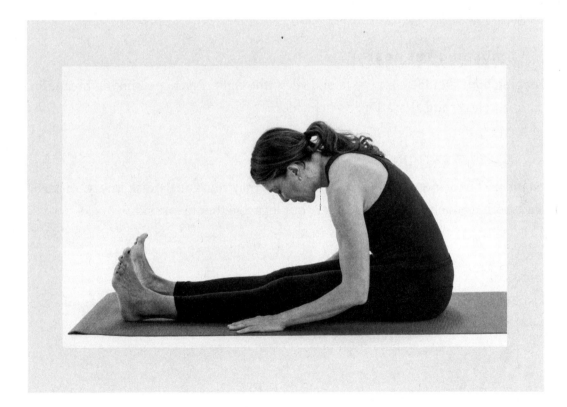

Lying Down Spinal Twist

Use this position to release your lower back after standing postures. It works well near the end of Mountain 3 to prepare your body for Final Relaxation.

GETTING INTO THE POSE

Lie down on the floor. From Knees to Chest pose, extend your left leg along the floor. Place your right foot on the floor and push to lift and shift your hips slightly to the right. Use your left hand to draw your right knee gently toward the floor.

HOLDING THE POSE

Keeping both shoulders on the floor, look to the right. Practice a sinking breath for optimal release and relaxation. Switch sides.

MODIFICATIONS

Caution: The rotation and flexion in this pose may aggravate a disk injury. Instead, place both feet on the floor and lower your legs together to one side.

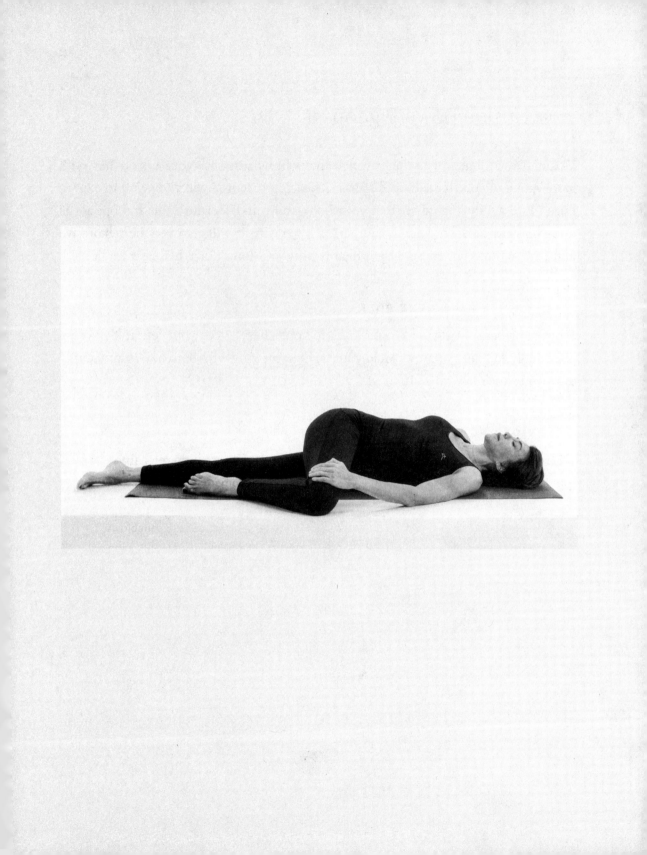

Upside Down Pigeon

Upside Down Pigeon is a deep stretch that will help release your hips, where you store much of your tension and stress. Releasing this area will allow you to experience more agility and balance in your body and mind. Because this hip opener is done on your back completely supported by gravity, it will also very be restorative and relaxing for your spine. Use it near the end of Mountain 3, before inversions.

GETTING INTO THE POSE

From your back, bring your right knee to your chest. Place your left ankle across your thigh and flex both feet. Hold your right hamstring with both hands and gently draw your knee toward your chest.

HOLDING THE POSE

With every exhale, continue drawing your knee close, focusing on releasing your left hip. Switch sides.

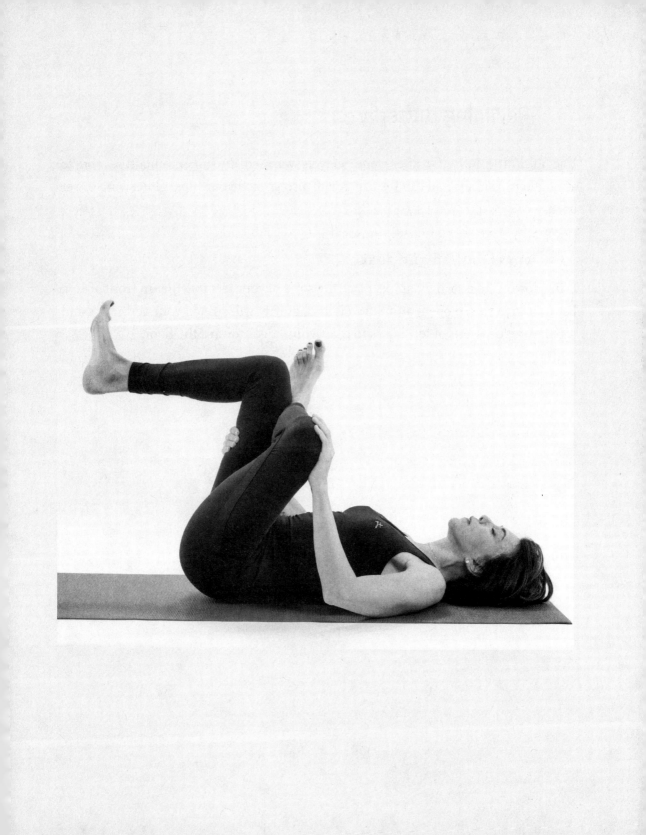

Reclining Butterfly

Use Reclining Butterfly after your body is warmed during Mountain 3, and to strengthen your abs and hip flexors. It will also stretch your hips, glutes, and lower back.

GETTING INTO THE POSE

Lying down with a straight spine, place the soles of your feet together in front of you. Let your knees drop open, and the weight of gravity will stretch your adductors and hip flexors. Use your outer thighs to draw your knees toward the floor.

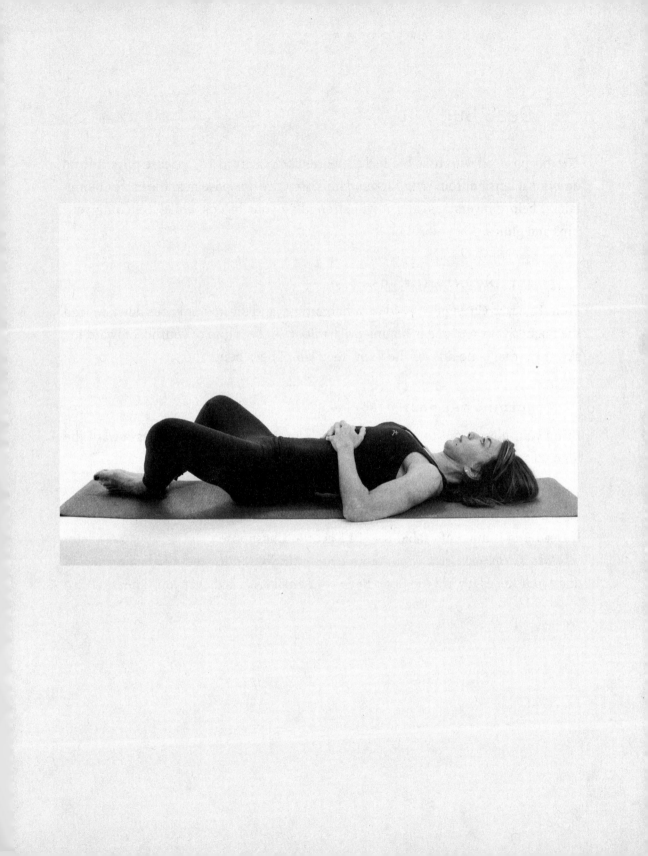

Dead Bug

For this pose, allow yourself to feel supported by gravity as you release physical and emotional tension from your back and hips. Practice this pose near the end of Mountain 3, before inversions, and it will strengthen your biceps while stretching your hips and glutes.

GETTING INTO THE POSE

From Knees to Chest pose, hold your hamstrings and draw your knees down toward the floor. If your tailbone is resting on the floor, lift the soles of your feet toward the sky. If your tailbone lifts off the floor, keep your knees bent.

HOLDING THE POSE

Bring your elbows out to each side; as you continue, draw your knees toward the floor. Rest your head, shoulders, and tailbone on the floor as you stretch.

MODIFICATIONS

If Dead Bug is uncomfortable, stay in Knees to Chest pose.

Take it to the next level: Grab your big toes with your index and middle fingers and draw your knees toward the floor. Keep your ankles stacked over your knees.

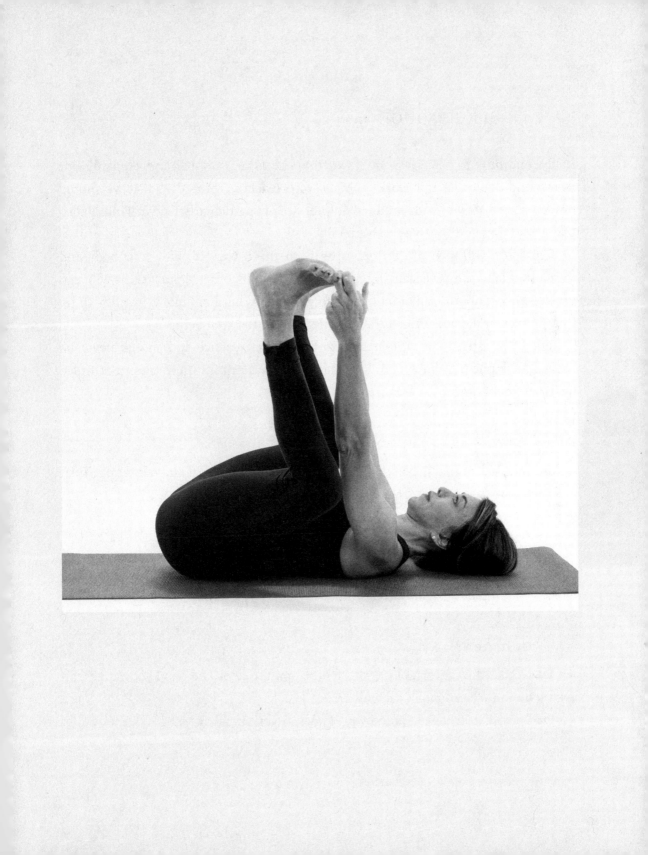

Final Relaxation

At the end of a YogaFit class we have completed our work-*out* and prepared our minds and bodies for our work-*in*. Many yoga teachers remind us that we should never confuse activity with productivity, and this is particularly true in Final Relaxation. By doing nothing, we receive plenty.

This pose will give you an opportunity to check back in with your body and mind, mentally and physically integrating the benefits of your practice. It will also provide an important transition back into your daily routine. Finally, it will help release muscular tension and stress for better health and well-being.

Final Relaxation is an integral part of any yoga practice and should never be rushed or skipped. At the end of Mountain 3, allow a minimum of 6 to 10 minutes for Final Relaxation.

GETTING INTO THE POSE

Lie on your back or in any position that allows you total comfort and relaxation. Turn your palms toward the sky and allow your feet to roll open.

HOLDING THE POSE

Let your breath return to its natural rhythmic cycle. Continue to release stress and tension, finding peace and calm.

MODIFICATIONS

For lower back discomfort, place your feet flat on the floor and bend your knees, allowing them to lean against each other.

Place a pillow or towel behind your knees or your head or both.

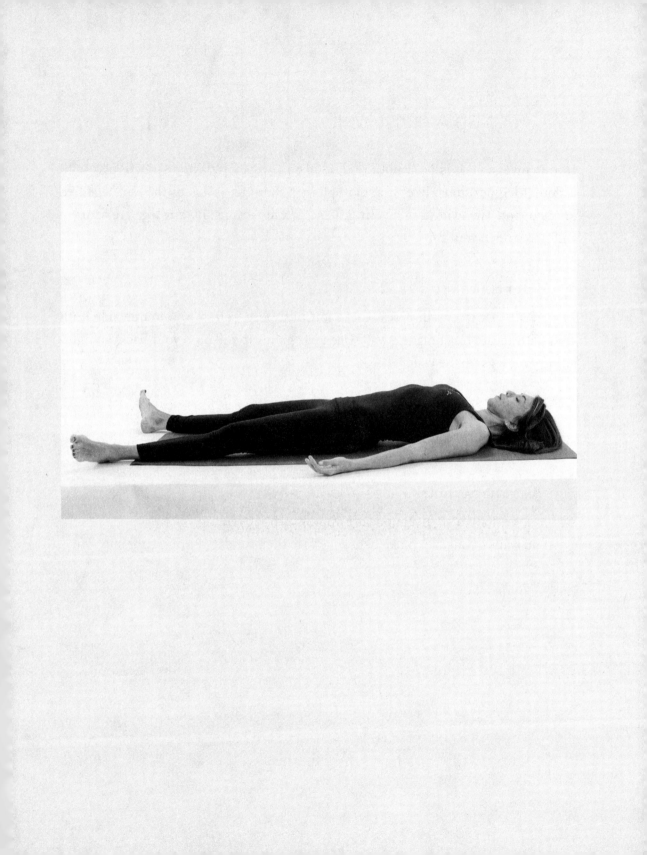

Legs Up Against Wall

In this inversion, it is hard not to relax. To add a deep, relaxing stretch, play with different leg positions, like Straddle Splits or Butterfly (soles of the feet together, knees open). This will stretch your glutes and hamstrings; if your legs are apart, it will also stretch your hips.

GETTING INTO THE POSE

Bring your mat to a wall. From Knees to Chest pose, roll over onto one side until your gluteals are touching the wall. Use your hands to roll onto your back, straightening your legs up the wall.

HOLDING THE POSE

Separate your legs slightly to breathe more easily into the bottom of your lungs.

MODIFICATIONS

Ask your doctor which inversions are appropriate for you.

If no wall is available, make fists and place them under your hips for support.

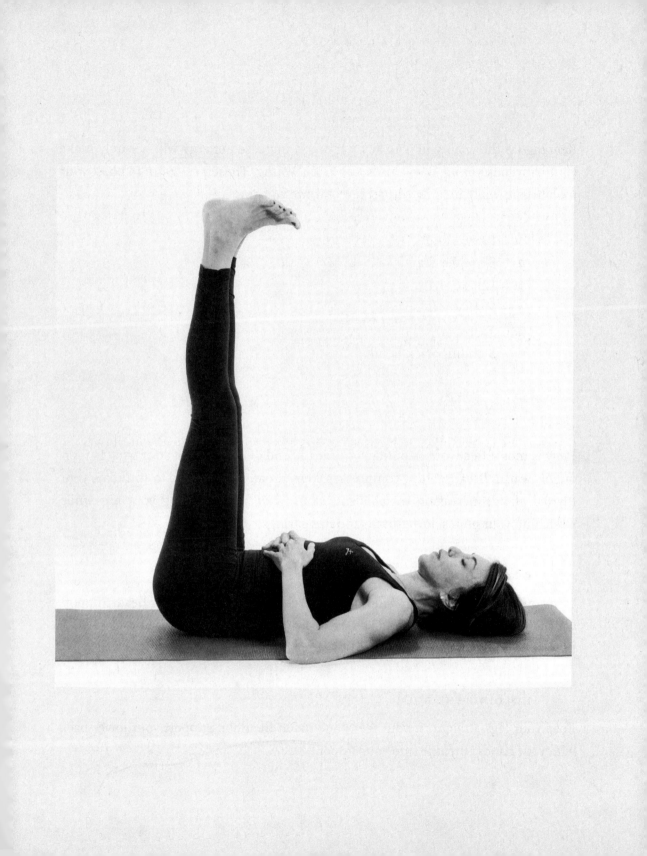

Anti-Aging

Keeping up the vitality in your body through increased energy will not only make your body look young, it will also start to feel young. These poses aim to boost your metabolism while helping you achieve a youthful being.

1. Plow
2. Shoulder Stand
3. Warrior III
4. Half Moon
5. Tree
6. Standing Back Bend

Plow

Plow is most effective in Mountain 3 near the end of class, when your body is thoroughly warm. Because Plow compresses your throat, it is believed to stimulate your thyroid gland, increasing metabolism, along with strengthening your abs while stretching your glutes, lower back, and hamstrings.

GETTING INTO THE POSE

Lying on your back, use your abdominals to bring your legs over your head. Support your lower back with your hands as you slowly straighten your legs and place your toes on the floor.

HOLDING THE POSE

Keep your legs straight. If your feet don't touch the floor, support your lower back with your hands. Breathe into your throat.

MODIFICATIONS

Reminder: People with certain conditions should not attempt this pose. Ask your doctor which inversions are appropriate for you.

Practice Legs Up Against Wall as an alternative.

If your toes don't reach the floor, place the tops of your feet on a chair.

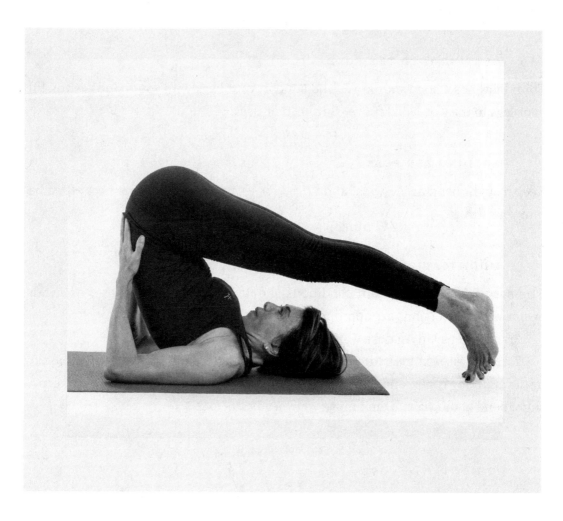

Shoulder Stand

Shoulder Stand is an inversion that follows the Plow pose at the end of Mountain 3. Like Plow, this pose is believed to stimulate the thyroid gland, increasing metabolism. Always follow with Knees to Chest pose, and it will strengthen your upper and lower back, abs, and glutes, while stretching your shoulders and chest.

GETTING INTO THE POSE

From Plow pose, bend your knees and support your back with your hands as you lift your legs to the sky. Don't move your head or neck.

HOLDING THE POSE

Keep a slight bend at the waist and knees for less pressure on your neck. Breathe into your throat.

MODIFICATIONS

Reminder: People with certain conditions should not attempt this pose. Ask your doctor which inversions are appropriate for you.

Practice Legs Up Against Wall as an alternative.

Take it to the next level: Straighten your legs and continue lifting them to the sky until your body is perpendicular to the floor. For less pressure on your neck, keep a slight bend at the waist. Don't move your head or neck.

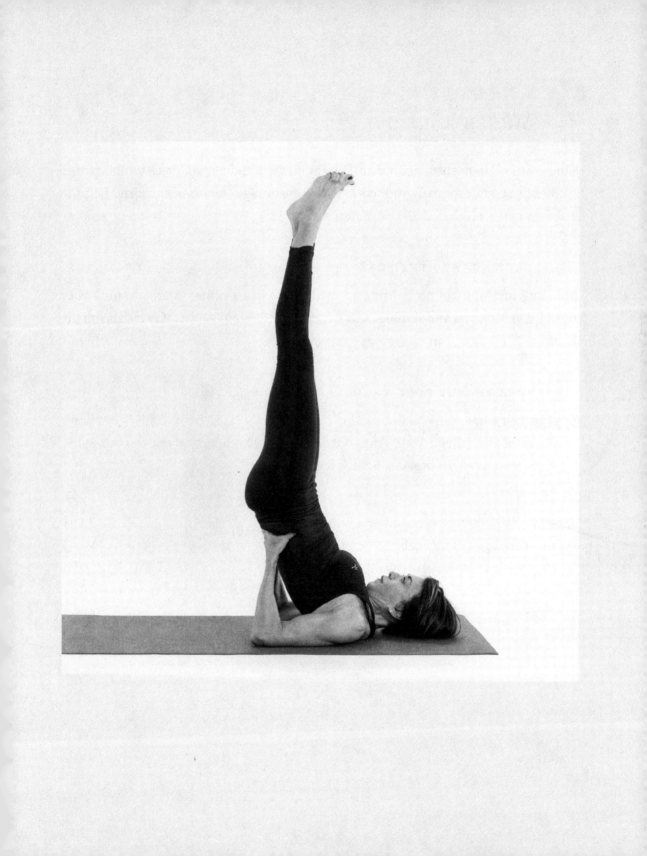

Warrior III

This pose will help strengthen your legs, ankles, shoulders, and back while it tones your entire body, especially your core. It also encourages better posture and helps to stabilize balance.

GETTING INTO THE POSE

Standing in Mountain pose, bring your hands to heart center. Start bringing your right leg behind you and tipping your upper body forward so that it is parallel to the floor.

HOLDING THE POSE

Engage your core.

If you'd like, extend your arms out from your shoulders or out to your sides. Hold for 10 to 20 deep breaths. Switch legs.

MODIFICATIONS

Do this pose against the wall.

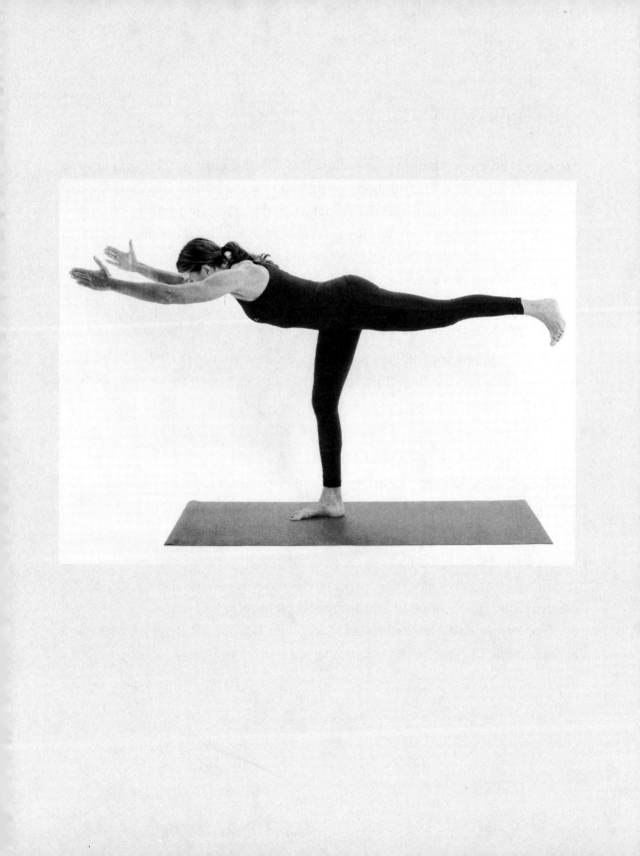

Half Moon

Half Moon pose is a standing yoga posture that will challenge your leg muscles and your ability to balance. This pose will strengthen your ankles and thighs, will stretch your hamstrings, obliques, and hip abductors, and will improve your balance, concentration, and core strength. While you will have the additional use of your hand in this balance pose, you will experience the added challenge of holding your spine parallel (or nearly) to the floor.

GETTING INTO THE POSE

From standing Forward Fold (see page 89) pose, raise your back leg level with your hip. Place your forward fingertips on the floor directly beneath your shoulder and your back hand on your hip.

HOLDING THE POSE

If balanced, roll your chest toward the sky and extend your top arm overhead. If you are balanced, look up to your top hand. Stay focused, breathing deeply. Switch sides.

MODIFICATIONS

If your hamstrings are tight, use a block under your lower hand. People with shoulder instability and rotator cuff injuries may want to avoid this pose.

Take it to the next level: Enter Half Moon from Warrior III. Bend your standing leg as necessary for balance and control as you transition.

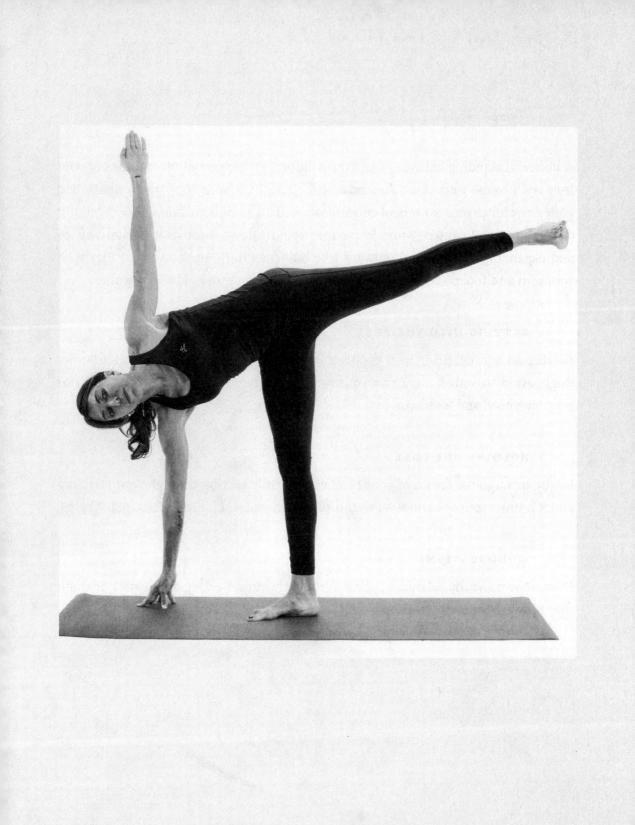

Tree

A powerful standing balance pose, Tree will force you to use all the muscles in your legs and engage your core. This pose will strengthen your legs, abdominals, and glutes as well as your powers of concentration. This popular balance pose promotes poise and calm. Visualize yourself as a tree, rooting down through your standing leg and expanding upward and outward like branches through your arms. Play with your arm and foot positions until you find a steady place to hold and breathe.

GETTING INTO THE POSE

Balance on one leg. Bring your opposite foot onto your standing ankle, calf, or inner thigh, avoiding your knee. Bring your hands into the prayer position, or raise your arms overhead and look up.

HOLDING THE POSE

Lift up through the crown of your head while firmly rooting through your standing foot. Contract your abs and level your hips. Switch sides. Finding a focal point helps.

MODIFICATIONS

If you have difficulty balancing, place the toes of your raised leg on the mat, or stand next to a wall for support. People with knee problems should use caution.

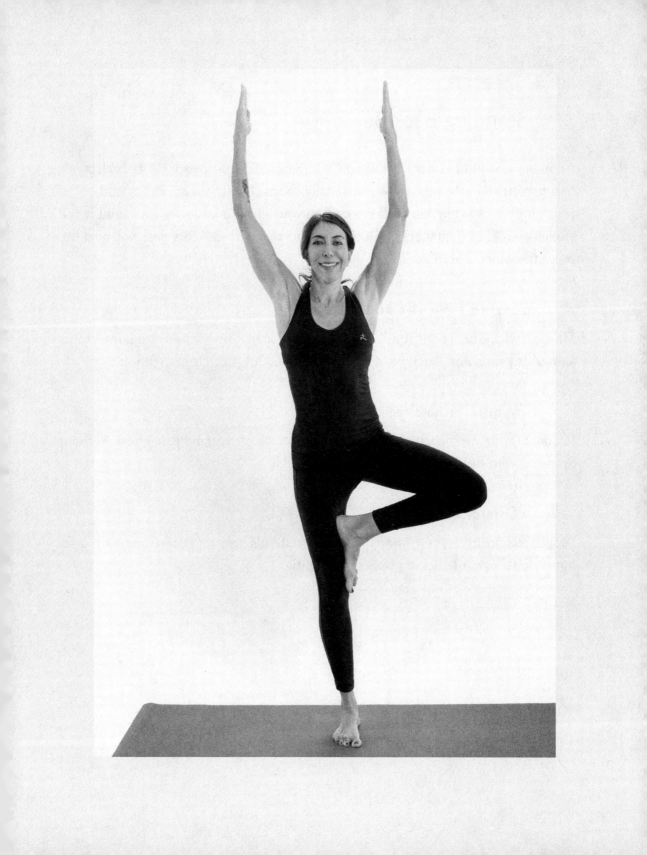

Standing Back Bend

Another valuable energizer, Standing Back Bends allow us to experience back bends in a particularly safe way, as you can really contract your glutes and extend out of your lower back. This pose will strengthen your glutes and lower back, and it will stretch your chest, shoulders, hip flexors, and abdominals. This pose will also improve flexibility in your spine.

GETTING INTO THE POSE

Move slowly. Firm your glutes and place your hands or fists on the bony points alongside your spine. Push your hips forward and lift your chest to the sky.

HOLDING THE POSE

Lift out of your lower back, drawing your elbows back to expand your chest. Without dropping your head back, look up toward the sky.

MODIFICATIONS

People recovering from a lower back injury should use caution. If your neck fatigues, look forward, tucking your chin slightly.

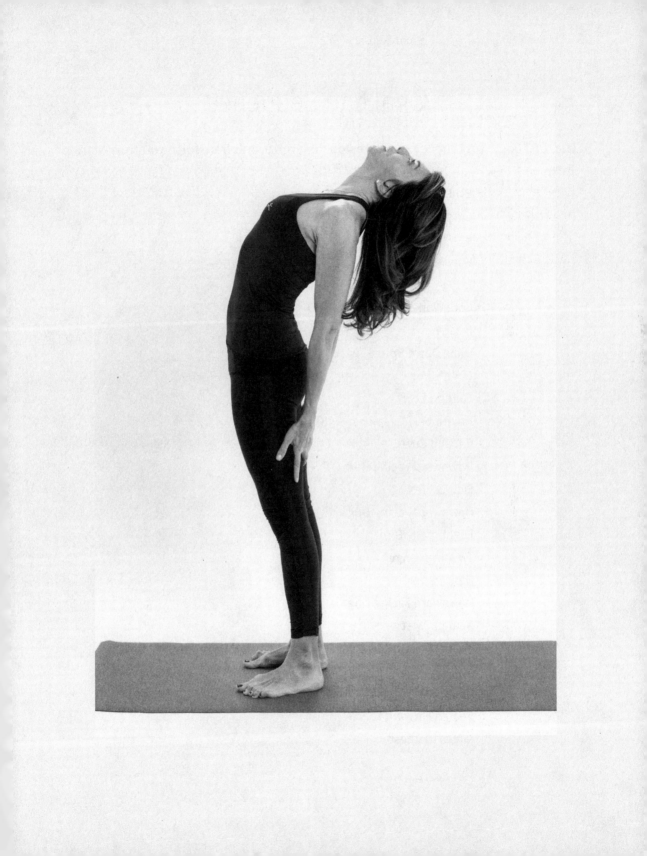

YogaLean Sequence

The total body workout below will restore, energize, and transform you from start to finish.

Bridge

Core Work

Bridge

Core Work

Bridge

Core Work

Bridge

Lying Down Spinal Twist

Child's Pose

Cat and Cow

Breath of Fire (see page 58)

Cat and Cow

Downward Facing Dog

Flow Series

Downward Facing Dog

Flight of the Bird

Twisting Lunge

Hip Opener

Downward Facing Dog

Seated Twist

Seated Forward Fold

Table Top

Boat

Seated Forward Fold

Knees to Chest

Dead Bug

Bridge

Reclining Butterfly

Final Relaxation

Relaxation and Rejuvenation

This sequence will relax you and rejuvenate your body and mind.

Knees to Chest

Lying Down Spinal Twist

Knees to Chest

Bridge

Knees to Chest

Upside Down Pigeon

Knees to Chest

Reclining Butterfly

Knees to Chest

Dead Bug

Knees to Chest

Knees to Chest

Plow (optional) *or* Legs Up Against Wall

Knees to Chest

Fish Pose

Knees to Chest

Final Relaxation

7

find your calm center— meditation

..

Beginning a Meditation Practice

s a child, I suffered from regular migraines. I would see beams of light in front of my eyes that signified their onset. These headaches were so profound that I would become nauseated. It was through these migraines that I taught myself creative visualization and meditation without even realizing it. I would lie down in the dark and imagine myself on a beach or in the forest. These visuals gave me an amazing space of peace and calm. As I got older, I tapped into that positive force more, and by the time I was an adolescent my migraines ended altogether.

I have been practicing yoga seriously since my early twenties. For many years, meditation was one of those things I flirted with but never committed to. I remember in my early practice I created a meditation "room" in my kitchen out of a trash closet but never actually sat in there, as it was too small. I meditated at the end of class occasionally, but never stuck to a practice.

In 2008 my life changed when I went to India for the first time. I knew I was shifting powerfully inside, but I was not sure why. I had a Vedic reading, and it explained everything to me, including the changes I was feeling within me and my past, and gave me a glimpse into the future. But what really changed me was that it made me become present in the current moment and realize that everything was okay. Veda, the spiritual Bible of ancient India, is a key part of yoga. Rig Veda, the oldest of the four Vedas, is where Vedic astrology comes from.

If you're interested in getting a Vedic reading, you can go to YogaFit.com.

Vedic astrology is part of the yoga tradition and operates on a different system than Western astrology.

In 2009, I entered my Saturn period, according to Vedic astrology; the Saturn period is a challenging one that forces us to learn patience and humility—a few qualities that were not exactly my particular strengths. Part of being in Saturn requires a consistent meditation practice. Meditation was always something I knew I had to "get to" but it was far down on my long list of things to do. Sitting still has never been my forte. In 2012 good friend and colleague Dr. Pam Peeke told me about Transcendental Meditation (TM)—she swore by it. I somehow intuitively knew I had to get trained in it. Ironically enough, I remember my mother doing TM in the late 1970s, but she quickly stopped, as she said it "slowed her down too much."

I dropped everything I had on my calendar for the next week and did the training. It was love at first try. I got addicted to it immediately—leaving parties to meditate, avoiding wine at social functions so I could meditate later, excusing myself from meetings to go meditate and return. I can truly say a regular meditation practice has changed my life. Despite running a yoga business, my life is very stressful: constant travel, businesses in multiple countries, and a few times a year traveling abroad to open the business in new locations, constant focus on the working of a business, opening studios in various cities, and managing some side businesses and family obligations. My meditation practice has become my "vacation" and my respite. It gives me the space to re-engage. I often will meditate anywhere between 4 and 7 P.M. for thirty minutes so I can recharge for an evening of business or social obligations. I also usually meditate for twenty minutes upon arising. I don't know if I would be able to manage my life without meditation, and I am so excited to share it with you. Where you go from here is up to you, but you just need to try it.

Since becoming involved in the yoga and fitness communities, I've had the opportunity to investigate the scientific benefits of meditation, and I'm happy to say that there's a lot of supporting documentation and research. People who meditate are able to activate the areas of true happiness and contentment in the brain more frequently and more intensely. Meditation also has several other physical and psychological benefits that I'll discuss later in this chapter.

So often I hear people say that they can't meditate because it requires an empty mind. The fact of the matter is that, in our hyperstimulated present, unless you live underneath a rock on the North Pole, an empty mind probably seems unattainable.

Much of our daily life is spent in our heads, focused on what we are thinking versus what we are feeling. With the demands of work and home, we are often required to stay one step ahead mentally just to get through the day. But if we navigate life by our thoughts alone, we miss out on a world of information available to us through our bodies. Meditation calms the molecules in our brain and body that speed around all day and crave food to slow them. Through meditation, we calm those molecules so that our body doesn't make us think we want food.

The ancient practice of meditation is as integral to yoga as the poses, with the same intention: not to tune out but to tune in to a frequency long forgotten—or perhaps undiscovered. Meditation is about becoming aware of what is going on within you as well as learning to tame your mind so that you can focus your energy and awareness on the task at hand. It helps you stay centered regardless of your circumstances. It doesn't teach you to avoid pain or discomfort but to experience and accept it so that you can move through any situation with a sense of inner peace and calm. Many different philosophies and religions say that the spirit is eternal, so we get in touch with the omnipresent through meditation. Eckhart Tolle talks about witnessing the eternal body; it's a wonderful way to tap into your internal "knowingness" and to get in touch with your essence.

Just like learning the breathing techniques and poses, meditation can be awkward and unfamiliar at first. It's eye-opening to discover that we are controlled by incessant thoughts and frustrating to realize that many of them are unnecessary and perhaps even untrue! Sitting in silence, we also realize how many common distractions compete for our attention: doubt, sleepiness, restlessness, and so on. Rather than using up even more energy fighting these hindrances, the person meditating eventually realizes that it's far easier to acknowledge and release them. Distractions will never let up, but we can learn to let them go. Awareness of our interior life and its distractions is the first step in developing a successful meditation practice that will improve our physical and mental well-being.

Once you get better at basic meditation, you can bring that focus into other areas of your life as well. No matter what is happening in your immediate environment, you can step back and respond, not just react unthinkingly. Whether it's an athletic competition, work, a difficult conversation, or just playing around, not only will we enjoy what we are doing that much more, we will do it that much better, too.

Advantages

One of the goals of meditation is to develop Lean Consciousness. In order to achieve any goal, you must consider where you are and where you want to be.

Most people have trouble with this because honesty is often a mix of shame, pride, resentment, hope, and criticism. Meditation allows us to activate the brain more fully and to find truth in our life holistically, even while it aids us to relax without eating.

Seeking Lean Consciousness involves a series of internal reflections from not passing judgment to being in the moment and honestly understanding our actions at that time. The depth of these reflections grows as we incorporate our new experiences and this new YogaLean lifestyle. If we don't truthfully establish our current state of being at any time, finding the path of least resistance to our goal (or destination) will prove difficult.

A shift in mental reasoning, while small, could be the boost you need to conquer your issues. For example, rather than accepting defeat just because you ate cake after dinner, cognitive therapy will shift the reasoning to a much more understanding one that accepts that you sometimes fall off the track but recognizes that that experience just provides another opportunity to grow. Meditation helps us integrate that way of thinking, acceptance, and forgiveness in our lives so that we don't dwell on a mistake or a hardship or something else negative stuck in our brains. It will allow us to honor those thoughts and let them go away without judging ourselves.

Scientific Advantages

In order to understand Lean Consciousness as a whole more fully, we first need to gain an understanding of the importance of meditation on a scientific level. As the different "spokes" of Lean Consciousness begin to latch onto your wheel, you will realize how much they rely on one another.

Meditation, one of those spokes, will help you gain an increased awareness and calm, allowing you to allocate your energy positively and to increase it overall. So often, low energy levels keep people from achieving their physical goals, but effective meditation will create that initial burst of energy needed to make a change.

CARDIOVASCULAR: The National Institutes of Health have granted more than $20 million to study whether there's a connection between transcendental meditation practice and the prevention or treatment of heart disease, hypertension, and stroke. Studies show that practicing mantra-based meditation twice a day reduces the activation of the sympathetic nervous system, resulting in dilated blood vessels and reduced stress hormones such as adrenaline and cortisol. Mantra-based meditation has also been proven to reduce high blood pressure, atherosclerosis, constriction of blood vessels, thickening of coronary arteries, use of antihypertensive medication, and mortality rates.

PARASYMPATHETIC NERVOUS SYSTEM: This is the branch that helps our body return to a calm, relaxed state after the threat of danger or even everyday stress.

When this branch of the peripheral nervous system is activated, the body can naturally recover and rebuild.

RESPIRATION/SLEEP/STRESS REDUCTION: Meditation slows down our respiration patterns, resulting in longer, deeper breaths, which, combined with the acquired ability to recover from stress naturally, leads to a better quality of sleep on a regular basis. You may find that you fall asleep often during meditation. This happens to me a lot. This means that your body is tired and that you should give it the rest that it needs. Many studies have shown that chronically sleep-deprived people eat up to 30 percent more food than those who are not sleep-deprived.

IMMUNE SYSTEM: A study at Ohio State University showed that relaxation techniques had positive effects on the immune system. The daily exercise of muscle relaxation was proven to reduce the risk of breast cancer recurrence. In another study at Ohio State, it was determined that a month of relaxation exercises boosted natural killer cells in the elderly, giving them a greater resistance to tumors and viruses.

FERTILITY: Meditation is good for the virility of both sexes! A study at the University of Western Australia found that women are more likely to conceive when they are relaxed, not stressed. A study at Trakya University in Turkey found that stress reduces sperm count and motility, suggesting that relaxation may also boost male fertility.

IRRITABLE BOWEL SYNDROME: Relaxation and meditation techniques have been studied widely, and their benefits can be found as a means to aid in large-scale or specific health issues. The State University of New York recommends meditation as a treatment for irritable bowel syndrome. When patients suffering from IBS began practicing a relaxation meditation twice daily, their symptoms of bloating, diarrhea, and constipation improved significantly.

HIGH BLOOD PRESSURE: Many Americans suffer from high blood pressure. A study at Harvard Medical School found that the effect that meditation has on high blood pressure is very similar to that of medication intended to lower blood pressure. They both make the body less responsive to stress hormones. While pharmaceuticals have been useful for many people, they also have their disadvantages, both financially and physically. Meditation costs nothing and has no negative health impact.

INFLAMMATION: Body inflammation, which is often caused by excess intake of sugar and/or stress, has also been linked to heart disease, arthritis, asthma, and skin conditions such as psoriasis, according to researchers at Emory University in Atlanta. Relaxation helps to treat all of the aforementioned issues because it switches off the stress response, allowing you to treat or prevent symptoms.

Mental and Emotional Benefits

To have emotional balance means to be free of neurotic behavior, which often leads to overeating. This is very hard to achieve fully, but meditation is one powerful way to improve such neuroses and unhealthy emotional states. As our consciousness is cleansed of emotionally soaked memories, not only does great freedom abound but great balance as well. Meditation helps with the following psychological aspects:

- Reduces anxiety and depression by enabling the body to balance its own neurochemical systems.
- Enables us to make better decisions and improve critical thinking.
- Breaks unhealthy habits by helping us detach the emotions associated with an action from the action itself.
- Improves communication with ourselves. When we better understand our own thought processes, we have more control over what we think.
- Helps us stay in the present moment. When we let go of the past and the future, we live 100 percent in the now, which affects all aspects of our lives and relationships.

- Helps to lower cortisol (stress) levels and to induce the relaxation response so that we are no longer dependent on food or alcohol to calm our nerves.

Executive Functioning

Mantra-based meditation has proven effects on both the brain and the heart. Transformational meditation provides the experience of "restful alertness," which reduces stress, strengthens communication between the brain's prefrontal cortex and other areas of the brain, and develops total brain function. What this means is that when the brain is focused or engaged in something, people who meditate regularly display stronger executive functions. People who have a high level of executive function have a tendency to accumulate traits that manifest themselves positively in many different facets of life.

STRONG EXECUTIVE FUNCTIONING

- Purposeful, flexible thinking
- Non-impulsive, proactive behavior
- Far-sighted decision-making
- Excellent working memory
- Settled, focused attention
- Avoidance of substance abuse or addictions
- Ethical thinking and behavior

HEALTHY PHYSIOLOGY

- Energy and vitality
- Fit cardiovascular system
- Balanced physiology
- Strong immune functioning

BALANCED EMOTIONS

- Self-confidence and secure self-esteem
- Feelings of safety and peace

- Compassion and empathy for others
- Healthy interpersonal relations
- Happiness and optimism

With a better understanding of yourself, the people in your life, and your world as a whole, you are then better equipped with the knowledge to make better short-term and long-term decisions, and the emotional responses to stressful situations will be much more balanced and appropriate.

Biological Benefits Relating to Weight Loss

Now that you've seen the benefits of relaxation techniques in general, let's talk about how they can help with weight loss or weight management specifically as well.

In 2009, the University of California, San Diego, did a study showing that, on average, Americans consume 34 gigabytes of content and 100,000 words of information in a day. With this much *stuff* bombarding our minds every day, we are always at risk for stress.

Just as relaxation and meditation techniques are widespread in their reach, so too is stress, but in an adverse way. As it relates to weight loss, stress can lead to impulsive, short-sighted, distracted decisions, like grabbing a Snickers bar because you're overloaded with work ("Hungry? Why Wait?"). Meditation allows us to hold true to our beliefs as we better understand their long-term impact.

Stress can also lead to physical issues like fatigue, high blood pressure, and a weaker immune system. Weight gain is often cyclical, but not as in someone who gains weight and then loses it will always gain it back. Rather, before accepting that one is not currently Lean Conscious, there's a cycle that runs like this: (1) knowing that a change needs to be made; (2) committing to making that change; and (3) postponing the start of that change.

It's not uncommon for people to resort to food during times of stress or discomfort. Some smokers choose not to quit smoking for fear that they might gain weight, figuring that the oral fixation that was previously filled by smoking a cigarette will be replaced with food. Before you can replace those harmful substances with more beneficial ones, you must first acknowledge that food is being used as a bandage for some other situation in your life. Ask yourself: Is this food or entertainment? How is this going to affect my body? Is this fuel or folly? Will this support me in my goals, or will it set me back?

Just by doing that, you have made the first step toward change. Next, it's time to evaluate honestly the various factors influencing your life. Is your job causing you undue stress? Make a note of that. Are your kids about to head off for college, and you're worried how an empty house may affect your marriage? Are you trying diet after diet to lose those last ten pounds but just can't get them off? Make a note of that. All of these things factor into your stress levels and also the manner in which you deal with stress.

Meditation offers the chance to focus on these factors and find their true place in our lives. You'll start to discover that what seemed like meaningless encounters soon forgotten may have actually been important touch points in your personal development.

Too often people find excuses to *not* retake control of their bodies. While some physical impairments may undoubtedly limit one's activity, I've seen things that seemed impossible with my own eyes.

Last year, I was on a flight from Chicago to Los Angeles when I was reminded of just how unlimited our bodies really are.

I had gotten settled into my seat while the other passengers filed onto the aircraft. I noticed that the woman who was about to sit next to me looked highly athletic, partly because of her matching Adidas track suit and her stoic physique. She admired and commented on my ring, which had a mantra on it. I asked her if she was a tennis player.

She introduced herself to me as Diana. Diana Nyad.

She was returning to Southern California from Chicago, after a trip to appear on *Oprah* during a media tour. Less than two weeks earlier, at the age of sixty-four, Diana Nyad became the first person ever to swim from Cuba to the United States, a distance of 110 miles, without assistance. Diana arrived in Key West after fifty-three hours. Even more astonishing than that was that she had tried it unsuccessfully four times before. When I asked her how she managed her immune system, she told me that she really did not do much of anything except listen to her body and eat what it told her to.

She did not let her age get in the way of her goal. She believed that her mind and body would allow her to swim through the Atlantic *regardless* of the year she was born or how many times she had failed before. She is a true example of the principles of YogaLean. I tell this story to enforce the notion that our bodies will go as far as our minds will let them—literally! Meditation will allow you to come to truth with your abilities and give you the mental tools to do what you set out to do.

Who are you and where do you want to be? Let meditation guide you to those answers.

Allow yourself to be a beginner. All you have to commit to is practicing, and your ability to concentrate will improve. Eventually, you will find that while meditating you will feel yourself slipping between thoughts, or you will be unaware of any specific thoughts at all. In this place, you not only tune out what's going on around you, you also will often discover that you've lost all sense of time itself. With enough practice, you'll find that you can meditate in a noisy airport or on a busy street corner without becoming distracted whatsoever.

Styles

There are four main styles of meditation: mantra-based, guided, visual, and somatic. They vary in regard to the senses being used primarily to engage in relaxation. Westerners live in a fast-paced society, and constant information exchange often benefits from active meditation techniques. Active meditation involves focusing the brain's energy and awareness on a particular thought or visualization. Choosing to focus the mind on something positive can help us to extinguish all negative thoughts and emotions. Whatever your meditation practice looks like, however, be sure to embrace the essence of YogaLean: Let go of all judgment of your experience.

Mantra-Based Meditation

Mantra-based meditation establishes a mental focal point. The repetition of a sound forces us to focus on it and, depending on what that sound is, we'll start to experience different changes in how we feel: Our blood pressure will lower, our heart rate will decrease, and our desire to overeat will also slowly go away.

A mantra can be a phrase, a word, a syllable, a group of words used during meditation, and within mantra-based technique there are main subsets: transcendental, transformational, and primordial.

Chanting is a great way to start your meditation practice. I like to chant along with my favorite chantress Snatam Kaur or Deva Premal. My favorite is "Ra Ma Da Sa Sa Say So Hung/The Siri Gaitri Mantra," chanted by and with Snatam Kaur. This chant is a great way to start a mantra-based meditation practice, and it literally saved my life during a very challenging time, alleviating a lot of stress and anxiety in connection to a very dark breakup I experienced years ago. It was the only music I could listen to for a month. It gave me a deep and profound sense of peace and calm. To this day, when I am stressed out and I feel my heart racing, I turn on this chant and chant along at the top of my lungs until I feel better. This music is truly healing on a cellular level.

"The Siri Gaitri Mantra" is a kundalini yoga healing chant that heals by tuning the soul to the pure vibration of the universe.

The words to this mantra are "Ra Ma Da Sa Sa Say So Hung."

Ra means the sun and connects us with that solar energy frequency.

Ma means the moon and aligns us to receive.

Da is the energy of the earth and it grounds us.

Sa is infinity and brings energy up and out, drawing to create space for the universe to heal us.

Sa for a second time, pulls the energy of infinity into us.

Say is a way of honoring the all-encompassing energy of the universe.

So is the vibration of the ultimate union.
Hung is the infinite, the vibrating real, and the essence of creation.
(So Hung together means I am Thou.)
Snatam Kaur's CD is available at YogaFit.com.

Transcendental Meditation was created in 1955 by Maharishi Mahesh Yogi, who began publicly teaching a traditional meditation technique learned from his master Brahmananda Saraswati.

TM provides the experience of "restful alertness," which reduces stress, strengthens communication between the brain's prefrontal cortex and different areas of the brain, and develops total brain functioning. As a result, the TM practitioner displays stronger executive functions, with more purposeful thinking and far-sighted decision-making.

Did you know? These celebrities love TM: Russell Brand, Jay Leno, Katy Perry, Oprah, Jerry Seinfeld.

Transformational Chakra Meditation is a YogaFit program designed to be a self-growth tool. It is a healing, anti-aging, stress-reducing technique that incorporates the use of mantra. Transformational Chakra Meditation uses the seed sounds, or bija mantras, associated with the chakras, the body's energy centers. This form of meditation gives us the opportunity to work on elements in ourselves that we feel need to be addressed and allows us to self-diagnose or take what we get from working with a therapist or coach and apply it to healing and transforming ourselves. It gives us the power and the opportunity to work on our issues as they are related to our chakras and provides a tool to facilitate deep shifts on an energetic and emotional or physical basis. We teach this at many of YogaFit's Mind Body Fitness Conferences.

Primordial Meditation (sound) uses a mantra chosen for us based on our birth information. It is usually a seed syllable that has a resonance with meaning when repeated. Deepak Chopra is an avid practitioner of this ancient practice of sound meditation in which you receive a personal mantra (or specific sound or vibration), which, when repeated silently, helps you to enter deeper levels of awareness.

Guided Meditation

This involves a teacher or instructor leading the individual or group through a journey, requiring us to listen and absorb what is being said, following his or her voice in guidance. It can help an individual discover hidden information, subconscious desires, thoughts captured from the dream state, insight to help make a decision, or techniques to induce a state of relaxation and repose. There is often a visual component or sometimes even a somatic quality to these types of meditation, depending on the auditory journey taken. Guided meditation practices can be helpful for beginners, as some people find them less intimidating. Other people may find them distracting. What's most important is that you find what works for you.

Visual Meditation

If you have to see something to comprehend it fully, no matter how good the verbal description is, visual meditation is probably for you. Or if you close your eyes and see shapes and colors or clear images, you too may have a propensity toward visual learning and meditation.

> For visual meditation, people optically focus on a given object with the intent to replicate the energy of that object. There are seven different subsets:
>
> **Tratak,** which involves fixing the eyes on something in the distance and not blinking. We spend all day looking at our cell phones or televisions or tablets—things close to our face—and this causes the muscles of our eyes to contract. Gazing into the distance allows those muscles to relax, restoring balance.

Palming the Eyes, while not technically a meditation practice, is an important adjunct practice for relaxing the musculature around the eyes and creating a situation conducive to meditation and overall healing.

Yantra meditation focuses on sacred geometric shapes that correspond to different energetic qualities and archetypal energies. The shapes are often from the yoga tradition and represent different personified forces.

Mandalas are another type of sacred geometric design and are often complex codified designs from the Buddhist tradition. Pictures of labyrinths can be used for gazing as well as complex imagery from Native American or other traditions.

Creating an Altar is a great visual form of meditation. Whether it is a collection of pillows in a corner, a group of candles, or your favorite photo positioned in front of your favorite chair, having a sacred place dedicated to relaxation is a positive and easy change to make.

Pictures, Images, or Small Mementos collected onto a board aid by placing images of positive things together, which marks that area for relaxation and positivity.

Statues can be represented by a cross, a Star of David, a figure of a deity, anything static and material. These can all be used for visual meditation practice.

Somatic Meditation

The prefix *soma-* refers to the body, and somatic practices begin with an awareness of the body. You can feel your body in space, notice a part of your body, connect with the sensation of how your body is sitting on the cushion or the earth, touch your skin, feel the wind against your hair.

Somatic practices can also be moving practices. Many people report that running feels like a meditative event. Tai chi and other slow practices can be moving meditations. Martial arts practices are moving meditations, albeit a bit more intense. Often surfers surf as much for the feeling of being immersed in the water and being at one with nature as they do for the rush of actually riding the crest of the wave.

Somatic meditation comes in three different forms.

- Eating is certainly one of the most somatic or body-oriented activities you participate in every day, multiple times a day. Make your food a meditation practice. Pause, breathe, center yourself, say a prayer over your food, smell it, thank it, taste it, notice yourself chewing. Slow down. Feel it. Before engaging in this type of meditation it's important to understand that in order to fully appreciate this method, you must know and accept food's place in your life. Healing the wound can't happen as long as there is a bandage of food over it.

- Meditation can also incorporate a mala, rosary, or worry beads. Using a counting tool or something to rub the fingers against helps to give a focal point for attention in both the body and the mind. A set of beads can help keep the count of a mantra during meditation if the desire is to engage in a set number of repetitions. It can also just be calming or soothing to engage the hands.

- Walking meditation is meditation while—guess what? Walking. Buddhist monk and prolific author Thich Nhat Hanh is a proponent of walking with attention and intention to make every step a meditation practice. You may find that when you meditate by walking you get into a flow state, because the repetitive movement stimulates relaxation and allows insights to come.

How to Practice Meditation

How can you use relaxation's healing powers? Harvard researchers found that yoga, meditation, and even repetitive prayer and mantras all induced the relaxation effect. The following steps will help you establish a personal active meditation practice:

1. Just do it. Commit to practicing your meditation for at least ten minutes (or however much time you have available) every day. It is help-

ful to set an alarm so that you don't have to keep one eye on the clock. To help make your meditation practice a habit, practice at the same time each day or immediately after your yoga practice. Finally, if you have room in your home, establish a special place to sit and meditate. Even if it's as simple as placing a chair in a corner near a window or surrounding a cushion with a few of your favorite candles, create a sacred space. Knowing you have somewhere you love to go will help you get there.

2.   Sit in a comfortable position with your spine straight, be it in a chair, on a cushion, or directly on the floor. If you are not comfortable, you will be distracted. If you are practicing before or after your YogaLean workout, roll up your mat and sit on it, as elevating your hips can ease tension in the hips and hamstrings and improve circulation to your legs while sitting for long periods.

3.   Use relaxation breath. Sitting upright with a neutral spine, relax your abdomen, and breathe quietly without forcing your exhalations. Take the same amount of time for both inhaling and exhaling, consciously beginning your inhale just as your exhale ends. The abdominal muscles must be unrestrained by tension or clothing and be completely free to move.

4.   Select one of the following techniques. If the technique you choose doesn't work, let it go and choose something else.

- Choose a *mantra* (word or phrase), thought, or feeling on which to meditate. Repeat it over and over in rhythm with your breath. If your first choice leads to negative thoughts or feelings, let it go and choose something else. For example, a commonly used mantra, "Om" (actually pronounced *Aaaaaah Ooooo Mmmmmm*), represents the root of all sounds that are ever-present as vibrations in our bodies.

- Visualize an object or place in which you find peace, such as a lotus blossom or a quiet beach.

- If preparing for a performance or competition of any kind, visualize yourself succeeding, incorporating all your senses as you mentally act out the scenario.

- Use a guided meditation. There are many such meditations available on CD. Relax and listen to each word fully.
- Use an affirmation card with a phrase that inspires or strengthens you. There are many books now available with positive affirmations as well as boxed card sets, or you can make your own.
- Focus on a small, meaningful object held in your hand or placed in front of you.

5.   When you're finished, journal about your experience so that you can keep track of your progress. For example, write down any techniques you tried and what you experienced practicing them. What were your thoughts and feelings before, during, and after meditating? Also, note if your practice revealed any solutions to questions or situations you've struggled to resolve. Finally, keep track of the benefits that you notice from incorporating meditation into your yoga practice. These will become incentives to continue!

Recognizing Your Success

How do you know if you are actually meditating successfully? Different people describe this meditative state in different ways. Some see a single source of light, some see themselves from a distance, while others see images or even sense colors. Some people simply see or feel nothing that they can express with words. Oftentimes you will experience a wonderful state of "beingness," an inner glow of warmth and peace. All of these experiences are successful. Just as there is no "right" version of a yoga pose, there is no "right" way to meditate.

As you begin to explore meditation and meditation techniques, remember that every day is different, every practice is different, and we are constantly faced with new struggles and challenges. Yet our inner truth remains the same; we need only look within.

Whatever your meditation practice looks like, be sure to embrace the essence of YogaFit and let go of all judgment of your personal experience.

I was blessed with the opportunity to have tea with Deepak Chopra recently. Eager to learn some of his methods, I was extremely encouraged to hear his words.

"I haven't missed a day of meditation in thirty years," he said.

While many of us will never achieve or desire that goal, meditation is a force in transforming, not just your body, but your mind and your spirit.

Try different techniques to see which one works for you and even if you don't think you're succeeding at it, do it anyway. Start by finding one or two ideal times per day and schedule around that. Then commit to thirty days and see if you can make a habit of it. As always, do not get down on yourself if you miss a day; forgive yourself and pick up the next day!

Tips and Tricks

- Use earplugs.
- Don't expect a clear mind at first.
- Breathe your way into it.
- Be patient.
- Honor your thoughts—all of them.
- Set an alarm.

The goal is just like an exercise—*just do it*. Engage in the practice and the benefits will follow suit.

8

cardio and weight training

..

as you've seen, Lean Consciousness is a state of mind that will help propel you toward weight loss and sustain your ideal weight when you get there. Achieving it, however, is not only about yoga and meditation. You must venture beyond the gentle, peaceful realm of poses, meditation, and breathing to do exercises that challenge your stamina and refine and build your physical strength.

Remember the wheel of YogaLean and its many spokes? It's not complete without cardio (aerobic exercise) and weight training because we simultaneously need to burn the fat off our bodies and keep our muscles strong and toned. Then yoga helps us stretch, center, balance, and focus. This creates a perfect trinity package of true mind/body/spirit fitness that keeps us in Lean Consciousness. Yoga and meditation without these last components is as incomplete as traditional exercise—running or lifting weights—would be without yoga and meditation! I learned this the hard way.

When I first moved from New York to Los Angeles in the early 1990s, I had a demanding job in advertising sales with a daunting commute that left me with little time for any kind of exercise or even much of a social life. I also had a boss who looked over my shoulder, micro-managing every detail of my day, and the salary hardly put a dent in my student loans and credit card debt! We've all been there, and it is very taxing on the body and spirit.

The combination of the long hours and stress conspired to pack thirty pounds right on me and all of a sudden I had zero energy and nothing to wear. I knew it was time to reclaim my health and power.

At the time, I couldn't find a yoga studio that opened early enough for me (5 A.M., yikes!), but since Los Angeles is filled with gyms, I found one where I could work out before braving the morning gridlock. Though I remember mornings at that gym as dark, there was a certain satisfaction in slowly getting back in shape and regaining my energy by using what I had time to do: cardio and weight training. I changed my eating habits—choosing hard boiled eggs instead of bean and cheese burritos.

I worked out hard and fast. I tore workouts from fitness magazines—workouts that got my heart rate up or that used free weights and Nautilus machines—and followed them strictly. In three months I had transformed my body and even felt a little elated despite my work/commute situation. People began to ask if I had a personal trainer!

If you think you can lose weight simply by lowering your calorie intake and doing yoga, think again. To burn body fat and maintain muscle size, we have to build our metabolism, a feat that cannot be accomplished simply by eating less. In fact, eating less usually decreases your metabolism and momentum without practicing cardiovascular exercise.

The Power of Cardio

The appropriate level of cardio is a decision between you and your doctor, but no matter what your threshold is, there are workouts that will meet your needs. Cardio exercise involves getting your heart rate up and sustaining the exercise to engage and strengthen your cardiovascular, circulatory, respiratory, and muscular systems to supply oxygen during sustained physical exercise.

It also facilitates the removal of toxins such as carbon dioxide and other waste products that are the by-products of dieting. Cardio actually increases the number and size of our blood vessels that supply our muscles with oxygen and nutrition. It also increases the total blood volume in our body. This means we won't fatigue as easily and can recover more quickly.

There is a wide variety of cardio activities to choose from, and changing up your workouts will not only keep you excited but will also help you avoid a plateau in your performance. Whatever activities you select should increase your pulse rate to the point that you are breathing heavily but could still carry on a conversation without too much trouble.

Adults should get at least three hours a week of moderate-intensity aerobic activity such as walking, or an hour and fifteen minutes a week of vigorous-intensity aerobic activity, such as jogging, or a combination of both. In addition, you should do muscle-strengthening activities, such as push-ups, sit-ups, or activities using resistance bands or weights. These activities should involve all major muscle groups and be done on two days a week, if not more.

I like to use this model of seven for weekly results:

> 2–3 Cardio sessions, 30–60 minutes each
> 2–3 Weight Training sessions, 20–60 minutes each
> 2–3 Yoga sessions, 20–60 minutes each

I know you are busy, so try waking up 30 minutes early and doing a 20-minute run or walk three days a week and do yoga two days a week. Getting to the gym may happen only on the weekends. Remember the effects are cumulative.

There will be some days that you combine both a cardio session and a yoga session and others when you do weight training session and yoga. That is what I want you to do! Seven times a week may sound daunting; start slow. Once you get into the swing of it, your body will crave these workouts.

Sample Workout Menus

"Any safe movement is good movement."

The best news is that you get to create a "Chinese menu" with a never-ending list of workouts to keep it fresh and fun. As we like to say at YogaFit, the one with the most options wins!

> The idea behind a "Chinese menu" is being able to pick and choose from a vast selection of options and combine them into your own unique "dish." Combining your favorite cardio workouts will help work out different body parts and muscles while keeping it fun.

Below are different types of cardio that you can incorporate into your training.

Walking

Walking is one of my favorite things to do because you can do it just about anywhere. If I have free time I will walk for hours, looking at flowers, houses, and my surroundings. For me walking is a spiritual experience and a type of meditation in which I can completely *immerse* myself in the energetic pattern of the location I am in and experience samādhi—bliss at being one with your surroundings.

BENEFITS

Walking can prevent or manage various conditions, including heart disease, high blood pressure, and type 2 diabetes. It strengthens your bones, lifts your mood, and improves your balance and coordination. The faster and more often you walk, the better.

GRATITUDE WALKING

Make walking an event you look forward to—an opportunity for positive reflection. Walk at a fast pace and reflect on the things in your life you are grateful for. This walk can be done anywhere—even in the gym on a treadmill. Here are some guidelines:

- Make it something special—I like to shower before my walk, put on my favorite perfume and a little makeup.
- Dress for the occasion—wear something inspirational. I am in love with YogaFit's tights topped with a YogaFit Tank or Burnout Wrap. (Always dress for ten to twenty degrees warmer than it is, because your body temperature will rise; if you are wearing too much clothing, it will be uncomfortable once you get heated up. If it's less than 40°F, you'll want to layer over your polar fleece tights. Whatever your choice of clothes, dress cute and you will feel better.)
- Wear a talisman—I like to wear a karma bracelet or something special given to me as a reminder of gratitude and good fortune. Accessorizing for your walk makes it meaningful.
- Bring a friend so that you can catch up—the time and miles will fly by. I also recommend bringing your best friend—your dog—whose excitement for a walk should inspire and motivate you like nothing else.
- If outside, bring your camera or smartphone—you may find little treasures along the way to photograph.
- As you walk repeat the mantra, "I'm so grateful, I'm so grateful, I'm so grateful for . . ." Acknowledge your blessings over and over again. Focus on the positive aspects of your life and the miracles that have come your way.
- Enjoy the scenery, clear your head, and *breathe* deeply.
- Do yoga, an inversion, or both when you return.

Here's my favorite post-walk YogaFit routine:

1. Knees to Chest
2. Spinal Twist
3. Core Work

4. Upside-Down Pigeon
5. Reclining Butterfly
6. Knees to Chest

Enjoy yourself and do it regularly—you can lose up to ten pounds in a month if you do this daily and watch your diet.

Hiking

I love hiking and do it often. Living in Los Angeles, I am blessed to be able to hike right in the city. At least three times a week, I take my dog to Runyon Canyon and we hike the hills for 45 minutes. If you keep a brisk pace, hiking uphill works the glutes and hamstrings, while hiking downhill works the quadriceps and calves. Hiking is one of the best ways to tone your legs.

BENEFITS

Hiking can help reduce insulin resistance in both the short and the long term. Hiking encourages healthy bone structure and reduces the chances of osteoporosis. Regardless of your pace, it will raise your heart rate and benefit your cardiovascular system, reducing the chance of heart disease and increasing your overall fitness. Being exposed to sunshine will also increase your levels of vitamin D.

Running

Running is one of the best ways to shed weight and tone up quickly. I personally have a love/hate relationship with running—it doesn't come naturally to me, but I love how it makes me feel. It gives my body a great workout without starting to break my muscles down. When in New York City, I like to run for twenty to forty minutes along the Hudson River.

Running is not appropriate for everyone. If you are severely overweight or have knee, hip, or ankle issues, it can be a problem. If you are lean, running can strip your body of precious muscle that actually helps your metabolism fire quickly, so start off slowly.

It is important to know your body well when learning to run. Go with your intuition to find your perfect run time to shed weight while maintaining healthy muscles, good posture, and a toned upper body.

Start slow and find your own perfect pace. Running is just like yoga—let go of judgment, expectation, and competition and run your own race. Running is an easy habit to form because of that addictive runner's high.

Cycling (Outdoor and Indoor)

If you want a fast burn, cycling is the way to go. It's more popular than ever, and the proliferation of indoor stationary cycling studios proves that this workout really works for people—not just physically but psychologically as well.

BENEFITS

Riding a bike is great for toning and building your muscles, especially in the lower half of the body—your calves, your thighs, and your rear end. It is also a low-impact exercise that is easy on the joints or those with preexisting leg or hip injuries.

Rowing

Rowing is a great way to balance out all the lower body cardio that you engage in. Most forms of cardio do not hit the upper body, and rowing is a great way to shift that. Depending on where you live, you can row outdoors or at the gym—most gyms nowadays offer stationary rowers.

BENEFITS

In addition to cardiovascular function, the benefits of rowing include increased upper body strength and endurance, targeting the major muscles of the upper, middle, and lower back and arms. Rowing also improves posture and increases confidence.

HIIT (High-Intensity Interval Training)

High-intensity interval training (HIIT) is a cardio training technique that alternates brief speed and recovery intervals to increase the overall intensity of your workout.

Most endurance workouts, such as walking, running, and cycling, are performed at a moderate/consistent intensity for a certain amount of time. For instance, you will work 30 minutes at an exertion level of 5 to 6 (on a scale of 1 to 10). HIIT is done at an exertion level of 7 or higher, and the intervals typically last from 30 seconds to 2 minutes, although they can also be as short as 10 seconds or as long as 5 minutes; the higher the intensity, the shorter the speed interval. Recovery intervals are equal to or longer than the speed intervals.

Here's an example:

> 30 seconds moderate intensity
> 10 seconds rest or low intensity
> 1 minute high intensity
> 20 seconds rest or low intensity
> Repeat the cycle 5 to 10 times

BENEFITS

The beauty of HIIT training is that you can get the same benefits as traditional cardio workouts in half the time. Keep in mind that this is high-intensity training; if you are new to exercising, build up the intensity slowly over the course of six weeks to avoid potential injuries.

Snowshoeing

Snowshoeing is an amazing workout and can be done anywhere that there is snow. I don't get to do it very often, but I love the feeling of going off without a plan into the woods and exploring.

BENEFITS

It tones your entire body while providing an excellent cardiovascular workout; it strengthens leg and heart muscles and improves delivery of oxygen to muscles.

Swimming

Hopping in a lake or ocean or doing laps in a pool will build endurance and muscle strength. Swimming is an excellent workout during the summer, as it will cool you down. You'll have no excuse to *not* get out and move.

BENEFITS

Swimming is a low-impact exercise that works every part of your body. It helps tone the muscles and is a perfect workout for those who suffer from arthritis.

Dancing

Engaging in dancing is fun and exciting, and it makes the time fly by. Whether you take a course at your gym, enroll in ballroom dancing, or just crank the music up at home and let loose, dancing is an incredible workout.

BENEFITS

The feel-good nature of dancing will not only lift your spirits but also increase your heart rate and allow your body to burn a lot of calories without you even realizing it. You will see weight-loss stories on *Dancing with the Stars* because of its great cardio benefits!

Weight Training

I've been lifting weights since I was fifteen. Weight training helps you build up muscle to make your daily life easier, increase your metabolism, and add more shape to your body. Weightlifting creates resistance against our muscles. Sometimes, when under high tension, our muscles become damaged at a microscopic level. The actual muscle building doesn't take place during the exercise, however, but rather during the recovery of those muscles. Weight training on a regular basis reduces the risk of injury, increases body confidence, and in general improves quality of life.

Muscle mass naturally diminishes with age, so anyone over the age of thirty really needs to start weight training. If you don't do anything to replace the lean muscle you are losing, you will naturally increase the percentage of fat in your body. Weight training helps you grow, preserve, and enhance your muscle mass, regardless of your age.

I love lifting weights and find it the perfect complement to my yoga practice. I like to do at least one or two sessions of heavy weights a week. The nice thing about weight training is that you will see benefits and results very quickly if you are consistent. It also makes you feel strong, powerful, and calm.

Weight training burns fat, creates definition, increases lean muscle mass, and burns calories more efficiently. It also increases metabolism by keeping more lean muscle tissue engaged and working. Think of your muscles like worker bees—the more muscle you work constantly, the leaner you will stay. Results will come quickly if you are consistent. You will enjoy noticeable improvements in your muscle tone, strength, and stamina in just a few weeks.

BENEFITS

- **Feel empowered:** Weight training gives you physical, mental, and emotional strength and confidence in your body.
- **Increased energy:** As you get stronger, you won't feel as tired or sluggish.
- **Anti-aging:** With weight training you can keep your body toned and tight into your nineties. Building muscle also contributes to better balance, helping you maintain independence as you age.
- **Build strong bones:** Weight training reduces the risk of osteoporosis. By stressing your bones, strength training increases bone density.
- **Boost your metabolism:** When you build muscle, your body begins to burn calo-

ries more efficiently. The more toned your muscles are, the easier it is to control your weight.

- **Manage chronic conditions:** Strength training can reduce the signs and symptoms of many chronic conditions, including back pain, arthritis, obesity, heart disease, and diabetes.
- **Sharpen your focus:** Research suggests that regular strength training helps improve attention for older adults.

There are two areas to consider when starting a weight training program: muscular endurance and muscular strength. Muscular endurance is how many times we can lift a sub-maximal (the weight just beneath the maximum weight we can lift) weight over a period of time. Not to be confused with cardiovascular endurance, which refers to heart and lung systems, muscular endurance is needed for everyday tasks like carrying objects around the house, taking out the garbage, and lifting the dishes out of the dishwasher. It refers to muscles we are using specifically to carry out the tasks in question. Muscular strength refers to the amount you can lift in one repetition or a maximal lift—for example, lifting a fifty-pound box off the floor.

At first you may wonder, "Should I do free weights or machines? Which is better for building muscle?" The answer: Both will build muscle, but free weights (dumbbells, barbells, cables) are better at doing it than specialized weight training machines. When we lift free weights, it takes a greater effort and more muscle involvement to stabilize the weights. The effort of stabilizing the weights also gives the smaller "accessory muscles" a workout, along with the primary muscle doing the work. Even lifting the dumbbells off the floor or the barbells off the rack will require a wide range of balance and stabilizing muscle to work.

With free weights, muscle effort varies throughout the exercise movement. A machine, by contrast, works the muscle with equal force throughout the range of motion, which is not as effective in muscular development. Free weights are just better at stimulating muscles, and more muscle stimulus means faster results. They also allow you to be more creative, as long as you are aware of proper form and body mechanics. Muscles love spontaneity—as does life!

Weight machines limit the muscle involvement due to the design of the machine or the singular movement pattern, but they are a great way to start weight training and get accustomed to weights while being able to maintain form and safety. We can easily hit all the major muscle groups with machines and strengthen our structure.

If you have to choose one or the other, choose free weights—they are cheap and easy to store in your home. However, if you have access to both, then take advantage of that and use both types. Muscles love variety!

Weight training: It works if you work it.

Since weight training can be done at home or in the gym, you have a few more options.

1.   **Body weight.** We can do many exercises with little or no equipment. Try push-ups, pull-ups, abdominal crunches, and leg squats. Many yoga poses actually force you to work against your own body weight. If you were stranded on a desert island with no weights or machines, your weight-resistant yoga practice would be enough. Common weight-resistant yoga poses include Plank, Crocodile, Sunflower, Chair Flow, and the Warrior series.

2.   **Resistance tubing.** Resistance tubing is inexpensive, lightweight tubing that provides resistance when stretched. You can choose from many types of resistance tubes online or in a sports store.

3.   **Weight machines.** You can find these at the gym if you don't happen to have one at home. Weight machines are a great way for beginners to get started as they provide structure and the possibility of good form.

USING FREE WEIGHTS

For the purposes of YogaLean, we will use free weights to engage our control and our core—the life force of our body's movement. You can use free weights or Body Bars, both of which can be purchased new or used very inexpensively in a variety of weights and sizes.

Before you begin your practice, I want you to remember that Lean Consciousness will teach you to appreciate the struggle and the opportunity to test and better your body through weight training. You must become comfortable being uncomfortable. Yoga regularly asks participants to contort into uncomfortable positions until the discomfort subsides—or, more specifically, until you can accept it and just let it go. Weight training does this as well, because although those last three curls hurt, the feeling of accomplishment will outweigh the discomfort.

One of the joys of weight training, and one that's heavily utilized in the principles of YogaLean, is that one's body weight can be used to improve that body, just as yoga does.

Listening to your body and gaining an understanding of your limits—these are very important when it comes to weight training. That said, there is a difference between what our muscles are "telling" us (as in, "Wow, this is hard work . . . so can we stop now!?") and what their message really means. For example, just because your arms quivered for the final three push-ups does not mean that you shouldn't find a way to still do them, because muscle growth and development come through exhausting the muscle first.

GETTING STARTED WITH FREE WEIGHTS

When you have your doctor's okay to begin a strength training program, choose a weight or resistance level heavy enough to tire your muscles after about 12 to 15 repetitions. Listen to your body during and after a weight training session. Although some muscle soreness is normal, sharp pain and sore or swollen joints are signs that you've overdone it.

After a few weeks, you should increase the weight or resistance, as you will be stronger and able to do more repetitions. I also suggest using the pyramid method, which means starting with light weights and then working your way to heavier weights as the reps progress. However, for the purpose of YogaLean, start with the heavier weight and, as you tire, grab a lighter weight rep by rep rather than quitting.

WEIGHT TRAINING PRESCRIPTION

I like to lift weights two to three times a week and work a variety of muscle groups.

Consistency is as important as is duration—ideally you want to spend 30 to 60 minutes lifting at least twice a week. However, three times a week is ideal, as it is for your yoga and cardio practice.

REST AND RECOVERY

To give your muscles time to recover, rest one to two days between exercising each specific muscle group. I find that I usually get sore 24 to 48 hours after a workout. I love the soreness that comes from a good weight training session; for me soreness means something happened, and it hurts so good.

In a typical exercise, I like to perform 4 sets of 12 to 15 reps.

Reps (Repetitions)

Reps are the number of times you will perform an exercise. For example, you will do 12 biceps curls and then stop. Each curl is considered one repetition. If you curl the dumbbell 15 times, then you have completed 15 repetitions of biceps curls.

Sets

Sets refer to how many times you will repeat that exercise for the set number of repetitions. For example, you will do 12 biceps curls, then rest. Then you will do another "set" of 12 curls, rest, and then another "set" of 12. That makes three complete sets of 12 reps.

six free weight exercises for the upper body

...

Rows with Bench

Shoulders/Biceps Push Press with Biceps Curl

Arms and Shoulders—V Lift

Dumbbell Chest Press

Overhead Triceps Extension

Triceps Kick Back

Rows with Bench

This exercise targets the rear delts, the rhomboids, and the entire core.

INSTRUCTIONS

- Place one hand and the opposite knee on the bench for stability. Hold a dumb-bell in the other hand.
- Engage all the muscles of the core.
- Bring weight down past the bench and then pull it up so that your elbow and wrist are in the same line.
- Repeat 12 to 15 times with a weight that starts to fatigue you around the tenth rep.
- Switch to the other side, placing opposite hand and knee on bench.
- Do 4 sets of 12 to 15 reps.

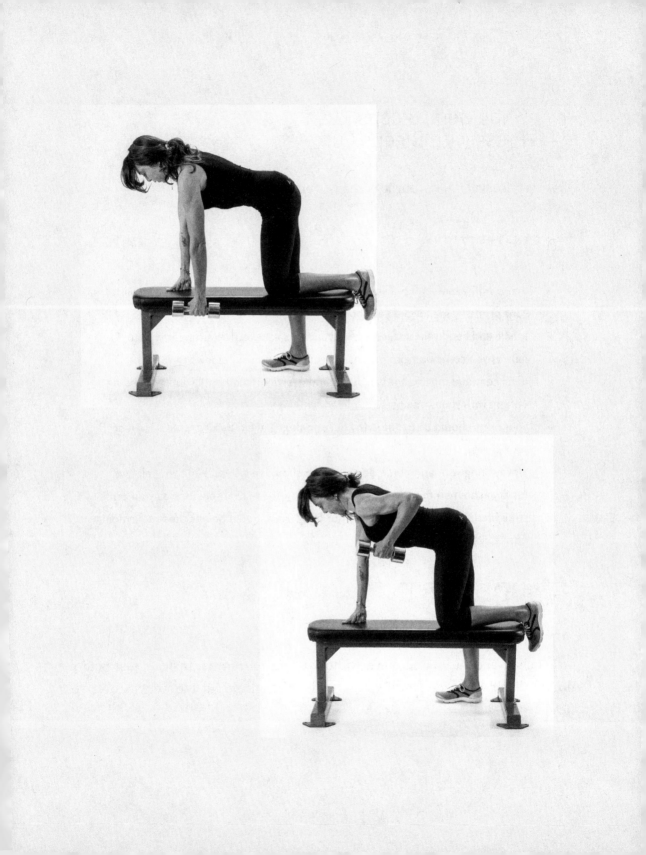

Shoulders/Biceps Push Press with Biceps Curl

This exercise will target your legs, arms, and shoulders.

INSTRUCTIONS

- Stand with your feet hip-distance apart, holding a dumbbell in each hand with your palms facing toward your body.
- Inhale and bend your knees and flex your hips as if you are sitting in a chair. Exhale as you come up from the chair position. Bend your elbows to your shoulders, continue moving the weight up and over your head until you are standing upright with your arms over your head.
- Your arms should be in line with your shoulders, avoid locking your elbows or your knees.
- Slowly bring your arms back down to your shoulders as you bend your elbows (as if you are hammering nails) and sit back into the chair position as your arms straighten and are at the sides of your body. This should be one fluid movement, from seated to standing.

Do 4 sets of 12 to 15 reps.

MODIFICATIONS

Use a chair and sit up and down without using your arms. Instead, just hold the dumbbells at your sides until you have the strength to lift the weights over your head.

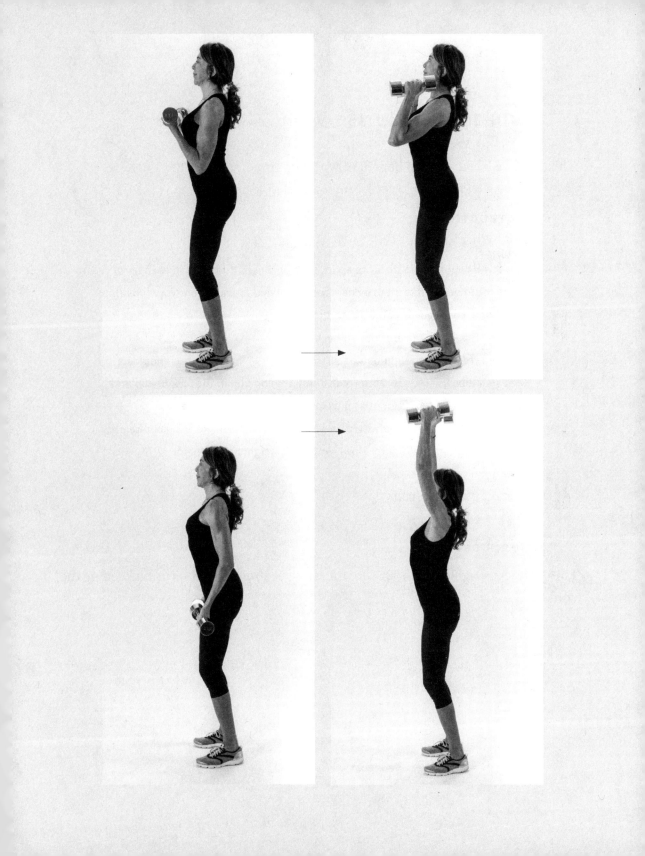

Arm and Shoulders—V Lift

This exercise has the added benefit of working the core.

INSTRUCTIONS

- Stand with your feet hip-distance apart, holding a light dumbbell in each hand. Bend your knees as if to sit in a chair and then bend forward from your hips (hip hinge) until your back is parallel with the ceiling.
- Keep your head in line with your spine.
- Let your arms hang straight down toward the floor in line with your shoulders.
- Keep your elbows straight. With your thumbs facing up, lift the weights up and out to the corners of the room as if to make the shape of the letter V.
- Hold your abdominals in very tight and only raise your arms to shoulder-height without swinging the weights. Slowly lower the weights and repeat.

Do 4 sets of 12 to 15 reps.

MODIFICATIONS

Eliminate the weights until your core muscles get stronger and focus on keeping the core steady.

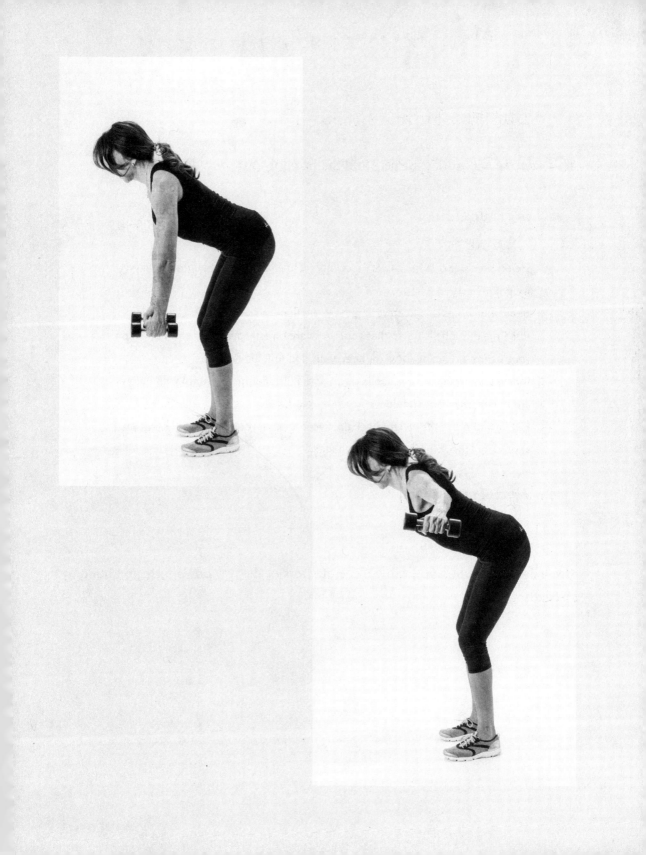

Dumbbell Chest Press

This exercise will work your pecs and the front of your shoulders.

INSTRUCTIONS

- Lie on the floor or a bench with a dumbbell in each hand; medium to heavy weight is best.
- Bend your knees and keep your feet on the floor or the bench.
- Push the dumbbells up so that your arms are directly over your shoulders and your palms are facing forward. Keep your abdominals firm.
- Inhale and lower the dumbbells down and a little to the side until your elbows are in line with your shoulders.
- Exhale and press the weight back up; avoid locking your elbows or letting your shoulder blades lift off the floor or bench.

Do 4 sets of 12 to 15 reps.

MODIFICATIONS

Use a lighter weight and go only three-quarters of the way down until you build up strength.

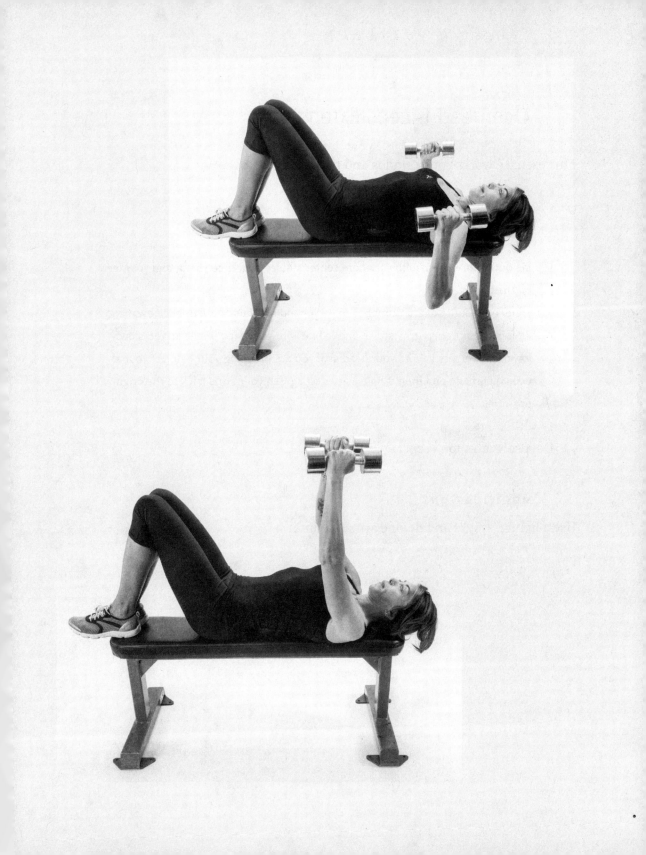

Overhead Triceps Extension

This exercise works your deltoids and triceps.

INSTRUCTIONS

- Lie down on a bench with your core center stable, your knees bent, and your feet on the bench.
- Hold a medium or light dumbbell in each hand and raise both directly overhead.
- Keeping your upper arms stable and in line with your ears, inhale as you slowly lower the weights behind your head as if you are brushing your hair. Let your elbows fully bend and then exhale as you straighten your arms back to the original position.

Do 4 sets of 12 to 15 reps.

MODIFICATIONS

Use a lighter weight and do one arm at a time.

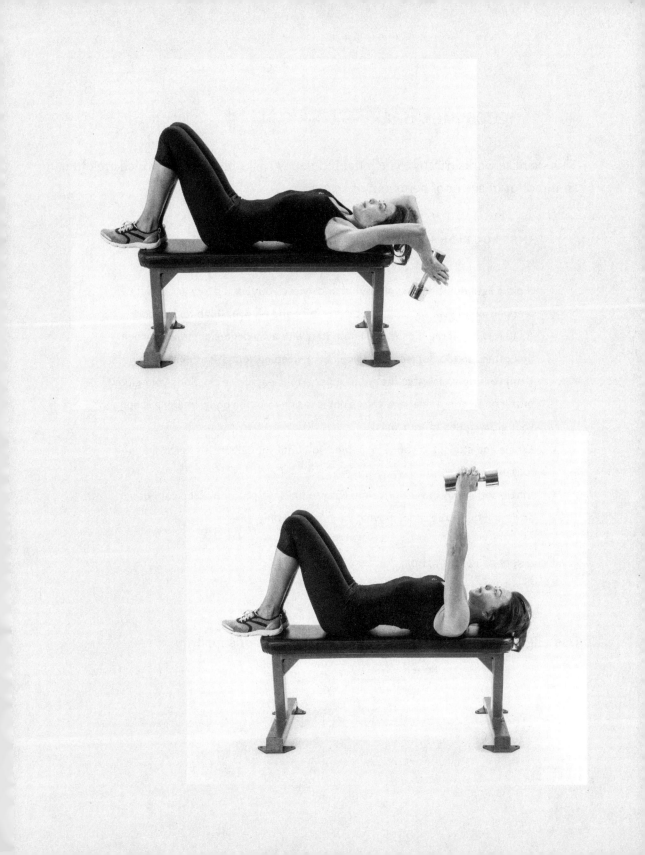

Triceps Kick Back

This exercise works triceps to help tighten flabby backs of the arms, which are often an indicator of age or of being out of shape.

INSTRUCTIONS

- Hold a light dumbbell in your right hand. Move your left leg forward about two feet in front of your right leg; place your left hand on your thigh for support.
- Bend forward at the hips (hip hinge). Start with a 90-degree angle, elbow bent, and extend to 180 degrees (a straight arm), keeping your abdominals firm.
- Bend your right elbow so that your upper arm is parallel to the floor, your elbow is at a 90-degree angle, and your palm is facing in to the body. Imagine keeping your elbow glued to your waist.
- Exhale and straighten your arm behind you until your elbow is straight but not fully extended.
- Inhale and slowly lower the weight back to the start position. Keep your upper arms still the entire time, moving your forearm only.

Do 4 sets of 12 to 15 reps.

MODIFICATIONS

Use a lighter weight and hold onto a chair or bench for support.

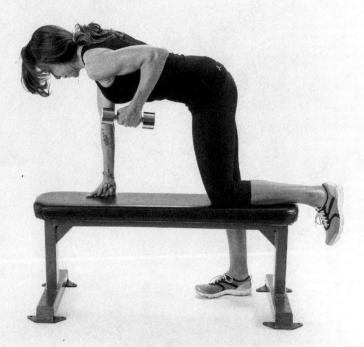

[modified]

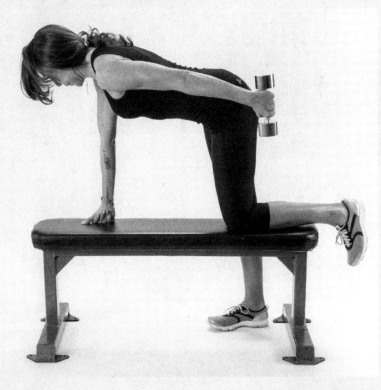

six free weight exercises for the lower body

. . .

Squat with Weights

Dead Lift (Bent Knee) with Weights

Chair Squat

Reverse Lunge with Weights

Side Lunge with Weights

Kick Back with Biceps Curl

Squat with Weights

This exercise will strengthen your thighs and glutes.

INSTRUCTIONS

- Hold weights near the chest, palms facing each other.
- Stand with your feet hip-distance apart and keep your weight back toward your heels. Hold your abdominals firm. Imagine sitting in a chair, inhale and bend your knees while leaning slightly forward from the hips about 45 degrees; bend until your thighs are about parallel to the floor, extending your weights forward.
- Exhale and return back to the starting position and stand back up. Avoid allowing your knees to move past your toes. Keep your eyes focused upward to avoid falling or leaning forward too much.

Do 4 sets of 12 to 15 reps.

MODIFICATIONS

Take the weight away and practice sitting up and down in a chair or bench to build up strength in your legs.

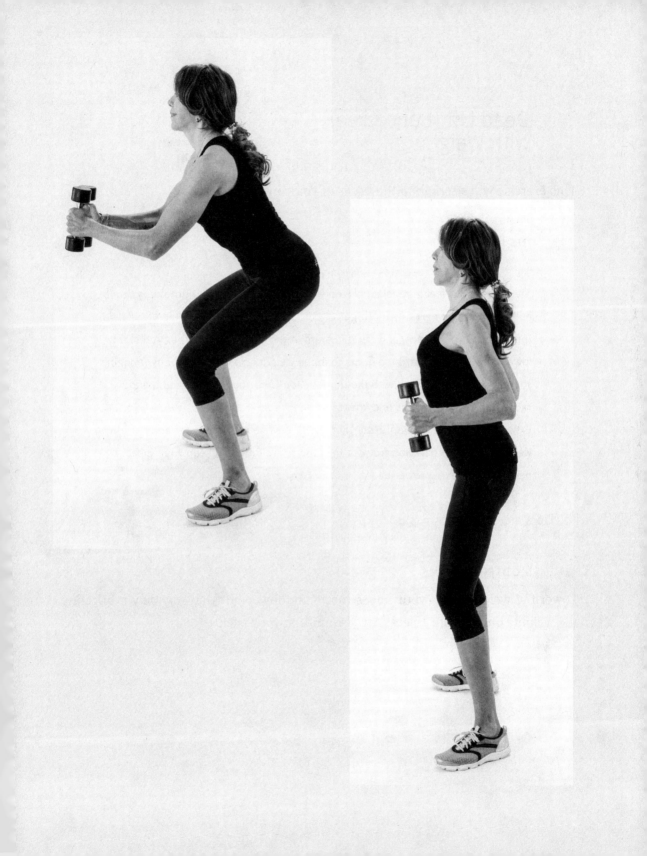

Dead Lift (Bent Knee) with Weights

This exercise will strengthen the backs of your thighs and glutes.

INSTRUCTIONS

- Stand with your feet parallel and hip-distance apart; hold a medium-heavy dumbbell in each hand next to your thighs.
- Inhale, bend your knees, and bend forward at the hips (hip hinge) as you slowly lower the weights toward the floor. Keep the weights close to your body (imagine you are shaving your legs with the dumbbells), keep your back straight, and move only from your hips and knees.
- Exhale and return back to the starting position while keeping your back straight.
- Keep your weight back toward your heel the entire time and keep your knees bent to protect your lower back.

Do 4 sets of 12 to 15 reps.

MODIFICATIONS

Lower the weight, bend your knees more, and lower only halfway down, bringing the weights only to your knees. Avoid rounding your back.

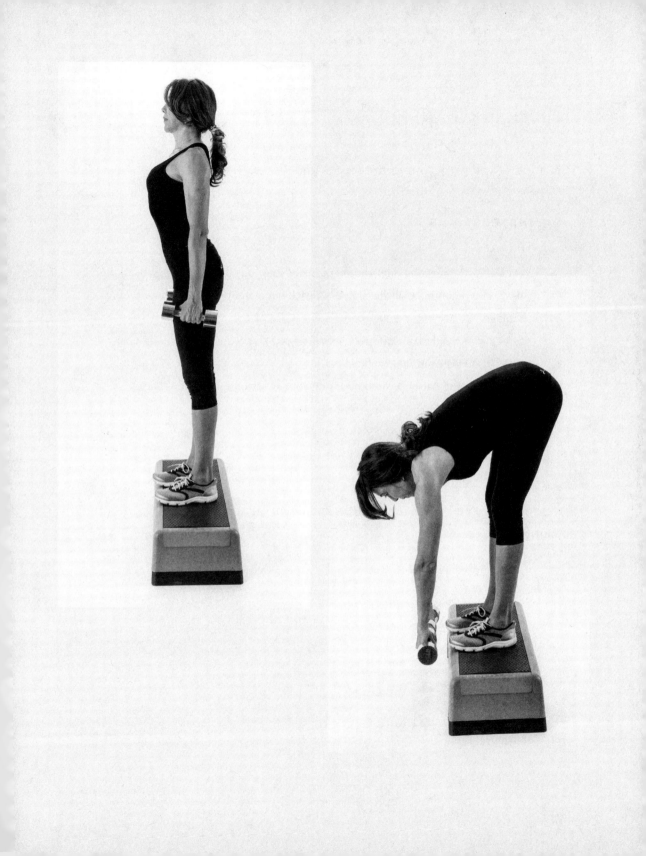

Chair Squat

This exercise will work your entire thighs and glutes.

INSTRUCTIONS

- Stand with your feet shoulder-width apart and your toes turned out slightly to the sides. Hold medium-heavy dumbbells in each hand and place them on top of shoulders.
- Keeping your weight back on heels, inhale as you slowly squat in a sitting position as if you were sitting in a chair.
- Exhale and stand back up without locking your knees or arching your back.

Do 4 sets of 12 to 15 reps.

MODIFICATIONS

Lower the weight and practice sitting up and down on a chair to build up the strength in your legs.

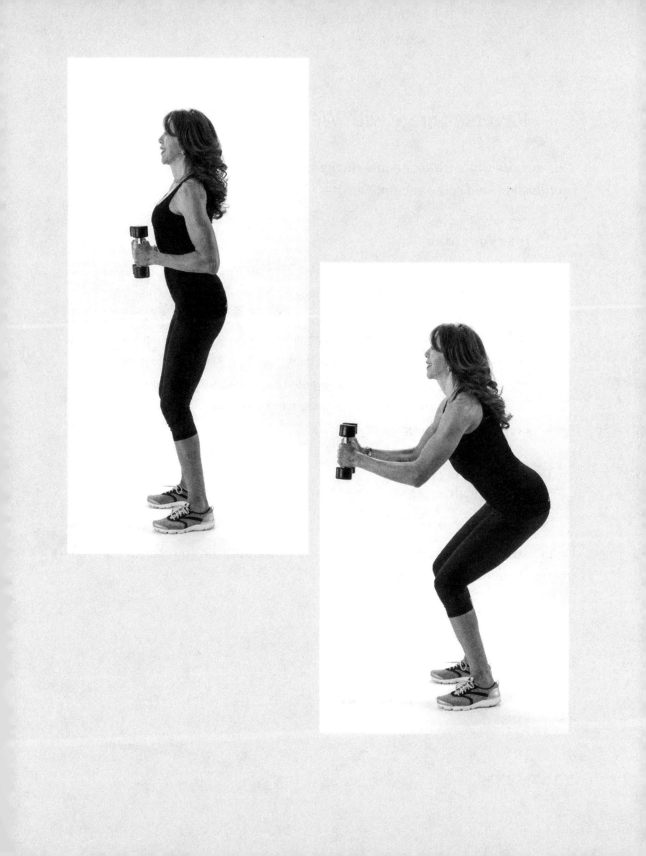

Reverse Lunge with Weights

This exercise will work your entire thighs and glutes and will improve your balance, coordination, and core strength.

INSTRUCTIONS

- Stand with your feet hip-width apart holding a medium-light dumbbell in each hand with your arms at your sides.
- Keeping your back straight and your abdominals firm, inhale as you step back with your right foot and lower your knee toward the floor. Keep your front knee aligned directly over your ankle, and keep your thighs parallel to the floor.
- Exhale and thrust your right leg back to the starting position.
- Repeat with your left leg.

Do 4 sets of 12 to 15 reps.

MODIFICATIONS

Do the exercise without holding weights and concentrate on your balance and controlling the movement in each leg.

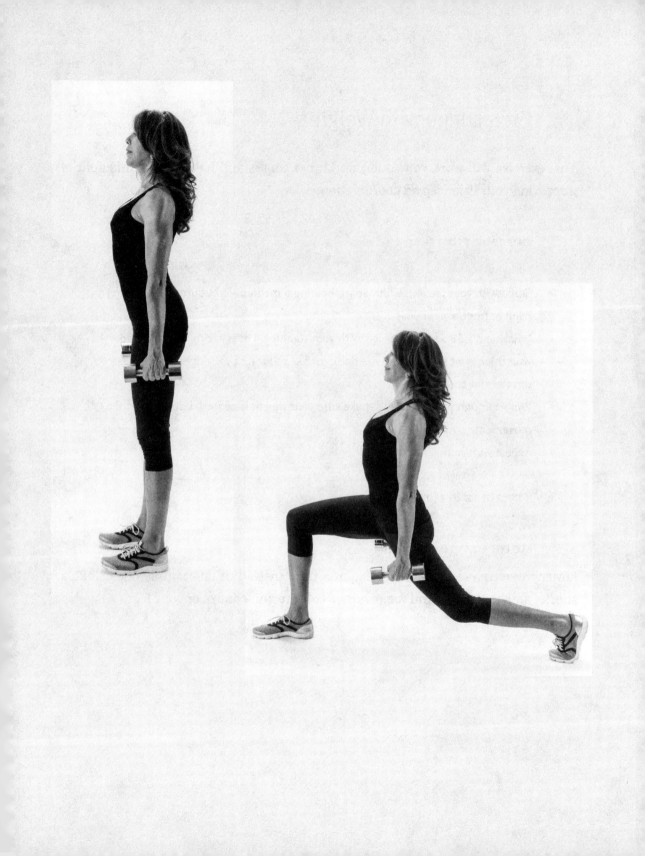

Side Lunge with Weights

This exercise will work your outer and inner thighs and has the added benefit of improving your balance and coordination.

INSTRUCTIONS

- Stand with your feet hip-width apart, holding a medium-light dumbbell in each hand in front of your waist.
- Inhale and take a step sideways with your right leg, knees facing forward, and your thigh almost parallel to the floor; exhale and thrust your right leg back to the starting position.
- Press through your heels and make sure your weight is centered throughout the movement.
- Repeat with your left leg.

Do 4 sets of 12 to 15 reps.

MODIFICATIONS

Lower the weight and work one leg at a time instead of alternating sides. Take a shorter step to the side and focus on the balance and control of your legs.

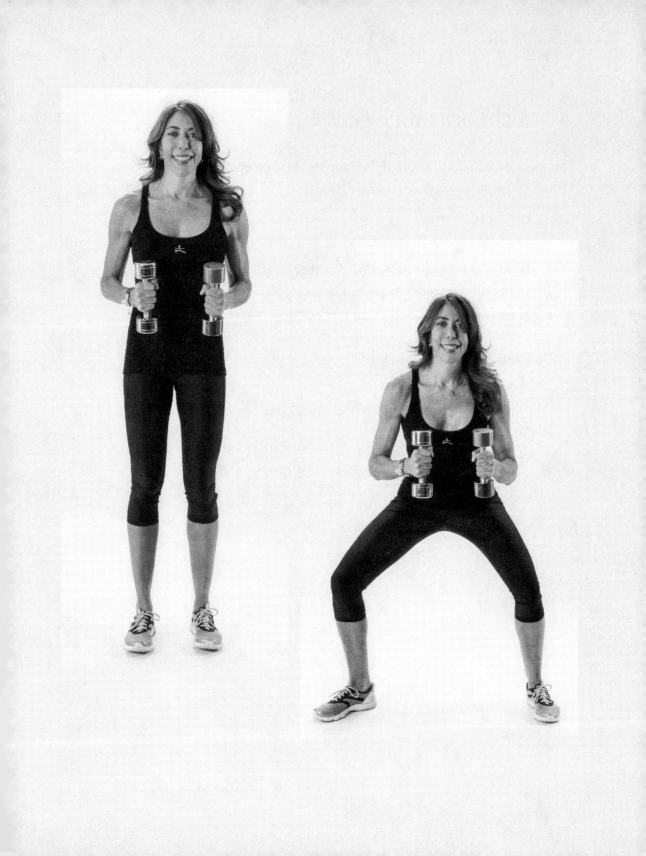

Kick Back with Biceps Curl

This exercise will build strength in your legs and biceps.

INSTRUCTIONS

- Standing in Mountain pose with a dumbbell in each hand, balance on one leg and kick the other one straight back, engaging your glutes.
- At the same time, do biceps curls with both arms. Repeat on your other leg.

Do 4 sets of 12 to 15 on each side.

ACTION ITEM

Utilize the YogaLean app for further step-by-step guides to yoga poses and exercises.

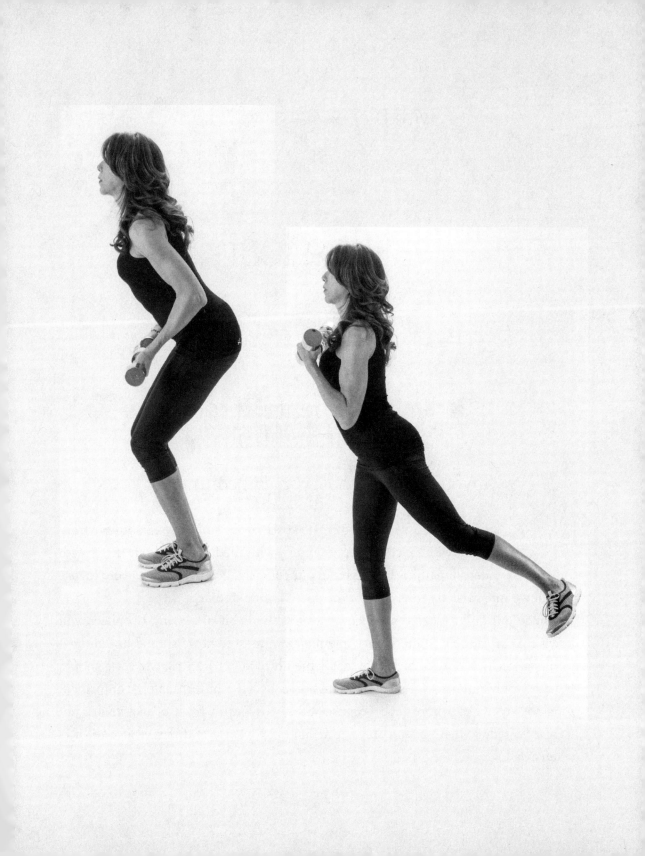

9

eating lean

..

Reducing Appetite Through Portion Control

"If you can stretch it, you can contract it."

We have discussed how to create space in so many ways, in our environment with de-cluttering, mentally with meditation, in our lungs with deep breathing, and even in our colons with a cleanse. In order to lose weight we must also be conscious of the space in our stomach.

Since our culture has developed an unhealthy habit of serving up plates and bowls that are double, sometimes triple the amount of food we should be eating—for instance, an 8-ounce chicken breast is the norm at restaurants, when we should be eating only 4 ounces per serving—our stomachs have, unfortunately, conformed. As a society, we eat more food because when it is put in front of us, we are not trained to reduce that portion size immediately. We eat it and pick at it until it is taken away.

The human stomach needs approximately two cups of food to feel full. Most portion sizes in America are 4 to 6 cups or more. According to registered dietitian Robyn Flipse, if you fill your stomach with more than that on a consistent basis, it will stretch out, which means it can hold more than the required amount. If you eat less, the stomach will do the opposite and will physically contract so that it does not require a large amount of food in order to be full, therefore you will become content with less. It's your job to sustain a smaller stomach size so that you don't overeat and gain weight.

Let's say you are already in the habit of eating 8 ounces of chicken at each sitting with all of the sides. You can start now and contract your stomach physically, which simply means feeling satisfied with less food. Many overweight people use surgical procedures including laparoscopic or gastric bypass to devise a smaller stomach; the hope here is that the patient will only be able to eat small amounts—but such procedures often don't work and are very risky.

So instead, let's look at ways to reduce the desires of your stomach and appetite by becoming accustomed to smaller portions and feeling hungry less frequently. Your body will start to get used to less and less food if you are *conscious* of when it is full. Tap into your stomach's internal compass, and feed it what it needs without overwhelming it.

Powerful tips to get YogaLean:

EAT BREAKFAST

Starting your day off with breakfast will give your body the fuel it needs to get going. Studies have shown that if you eat breakfast, you will also snack less throughout the day. Adding protein to your meal will give you added energy.

DRINK WATER

The first thing you should do every morning is drink a tall glass of water. This awakens your internal organs and hydrates you after eight hours of dehydration (if you're getting enough sleep, that is). Throughout the day, drink constantly and make sure you get at least eight 8-ounce glasses in; water helps you feel full.

To help save the environment from excess plastic bottles, get a Brita pitcher. That way, you can save money and the earth at the same time.

FIBER AND WHOLE GRAINS!

Incorporating fiber and whole grains into meals will keep you fuller longer. Try an apple with almonds—my favorite high-fiber and energetic snack in between meals.

RECOGNIZE THE FEELING OF HUNGER

"Just because you can does not mean you have to."

If you're not hungry, don't eat. Tap into your Lean Consciousness and eat only when you're hungry, not when you're bored, sad, stressed, or socializing. Listen to your body and begin to know when you *need* to eat rather than when you *want* to!

REDUCE YOUR PLATE SIZE AND YOUR FORK SIZE

We eat with our eyes; when our plate is full, our eyes will want to eat everything on the plate. A great fix to this is serving your meals on smaller plates and eating with a smaller fork or with chopsticks. Seeing a huge plate that's only partially filled will make you feel like you're missing something, so feel your (smaller) plate and feast (with your eyes too).

PORTION CONTROL

Remember my friend who, before eating, split her meal in half and stored the rest for leftovers? I want you to do the same. It's like that classic fashion tip—before going out, look in the mirror and remove two accessories. This applies to your meals as well—look at the massive plate you are used to eating, then divide it in half or in thirds and practice eating smaller, more frequent meals. Try ordering appetizers or sides instead of the main course.

BREATHE

Enjoy your food and the time you spend eating it! Eat slowly, and give your body proper time to digest. It takes your body twenty to thirty minutes to recognize when you're full. If you eat like you're in a race, your body doesn't register how much you've eaten until it's too late. Slowing down allows yourself to notice and *feel* when you are full.

FEEL SATISFIED, NOT FULL

Practice leaving the table slightly hungry—remember that it takes twenty to thirty minutes for the stomach to send the signal to the brain that it's full. Avoid leaving the table completely and utterly full. In fact, leave your stomach a little breathing room so that you don't feel bogged down.

GET RID OF SNACKS/JUNK FOOD

You will not eat food that is not there to begin with, so don't have bad food in your house or in your desk at work. If you keep food elsewhere, you will have to work to get it, which will allow you time to think before mindlessly doing it.

PORTION OUT FOOD BEFORE EATING

Don't eat straight out of the package. Measure out cereal, brown rice, berries, and other foods before eating, then put the rest away. Doing this will give you an exact visual of how much you should be eating, and this will help you avoid overeating. Use a scale if necessary.

Eating Clean

Once you cultivate a regular yoga practice, you will notice a change for the better. Within weeks you will feel lighter, physically and mentally. As you begin to develop body awareness, you will notice your food choices change; you will start to crave healthier, more organic food. No longer will you want to fill your body with processed foods, fatty meats, and sugary, carbohydrate-laden items. You may even shy away from caffeine and alcohol. When you get in touch with your body, you can then listen to the messages it sends you—your body doesn't want junk, packaged, or fast food. Food is fuel. Your body, on a cellular level, wants fresh healthy foods, primarily fruits and vegetables, whole grains, and legumes.

YogaLean focuses on building a relationship with supportive foods and drinks that support your body's functioning and banishing destructive foods that are hurting you. This program eliminates gluten, white flour, sugar, processed foods, and excess meat from your diet so that you will feel lighter and healthier. Your food cravings will begin to dissipate, and you will feel an overall sense of balance simply from that shift in nutrition. While "diets" don't typically work in the long run, YogaLean places enormous emphasis on good nutrition and an overall change in the way you look at food and how it affects your body.

Eating clean is a huge aspect of gaining Lean Consciousness. It's not a diet; rather, it's about putting an effort into the foods we purchase and incorporate into our meals and giving our bodies the nutrients they need to maintain a high level of productivity. Essentially, this means abolishing pesticides, additives, preservatives, artificial sweeteners, gluten, and other chemicals from our diet and sticking to the earth's natural foods—organic veggies and fruits, wild-caught fish, whole grains, natural sweeteners, legumes, and nuts.

Even if you want to lose only five pounds, poor nutrition is impacting your health in untold ways. There is absolute truth to the adage "You are what you eat," and unfortunately, our bodies are bombarded with unnatural chemicals and additives that are affecting every aspect of our lives and well-being, including increased risk for diseases, sickness, and cancer. The good news is that we can choose what goes into our bodies and begin to lose weight and improve our health in real time, with just a few simple changes. While weight loss should be slow and gradual, as soon as you take the action to eat clean, you will likely notice increased energy, mental clarity, and a more positive attitude—all of which make it easier to exercise, avoid binges, practice the yamas and niyamas, and generally move from stagnation to celebration on a daily basis.

As you begin to eat better, your body will begin to burn fat more efficiently, recognize once again when you are hungry and full, clear the clutter that decreases your health, release toxins stored in the abdominal area, improve cholesterol ratios, decrease inflammation, lower blood sugar levels, and lower blood pressure. By reversing these conditions, you greatly improve your chances of avoiding everything from cardiovascular disease and cancer to diabetes and Alzheimer's disease. It's worth it!

In the morning we turn to caffeine for energy, only to relax with alcohol at night. Not only can these habits make us fat, they dramatically impact our brains, decrease our libidos, alter our appearance (skin, hair, and so on), confuse and damage our endocrine systems (hormones), and accelerate the aging process. Furthermore, diet can significantly affect mood, even leading to depression, which alters eating and exercise habits and ends up creating a vicious cycle that makes weight loss nearly impossible.

When you are in the grocery store, pay attention the labels, and by that I mean look at the list of ingredients and envision those words going into your body. If it says "fat free," oftentimes the producer will replace the fat with additives so that it still tastes good (and seems "healthy"). The abundance of fat-free and sugar-free products on the market has confused the issue of how to control weight and stay healthy—just because it says "fat free" doesn't mean it's healthy (Sour Patch Kids are "fat free," after all); just because it says "sugar free" doesn't mean it's not riddled with other chemicals that make it taste like sugar. Furthermore, vegan "chicken" goes through a very rigorous process to make it imitate chicken, so just because it says "vegan" doesn't mean it's clean.

Also, learn portion and serving size. If the label says "serving size ¼ cup," then measure a quarter cup and eat only that much per serving.

Organic Food

For many people, traveling internationally is an introduction to actual fresh food—or, as they call it in much of the rest of the world, "food"! This is not to say you cannot access delicious nonprocessed foods in the United States; you just may have to make a little bit more of an effort. I try to go to a farmers' market weekly.

"Organic" refers to how farmers grow and process their fruits, vegetables, meats, dairy, and grains. Instead of using chemicals to aid in the growth and protection of their agriculture, they embrace natural methods. For instance, rather than spraying their produce with pesticides or expediting its growth through fertilizer, they will use a knowledge of different types of soil, water conservation, and other techniques to reduce the impact of chemicals on the food.

Organic food is often more expensive than conventionally grown items, so here are a few rules to know when it's truly worth it. When buying produce, it's important to go organic with items with thin/exposed skin, as they hold on to the most pesticide residue. They might look odd shaped or imperfect, but enter the produce aisle with nonjudgment in mind:

- Apples
- Cherries
- Berries
- Grapes
- Nectarines
- Peaches
- Pears
- Bell peppers
- Celery
- Greens (lettuces, spinach, kale, chard, etc.)
- Potatoes

All meats and dairy should be organic, free-range, cruelty-free, hormone-free, grass-fed.

Wild-Caught Fish

This is what it means to be a "farm raised" fish: The producer gathers all the little fish and stores them in a huge tank with all of the other little fish. The producer then continues to pack the tank until it becomes more crowded. These fish begin to eat each other's waste, filling their bodies with grime and other toxins, which we then consume at home. Get to know the guy (or gal) behind the fish counter. Look for the "wild caught" label and purchase what's in season!

GOOD ALL YEAR LONG
- Ahi tuna
- Cod
- Sole
- Mahimahi
- Atlantic salmon
- Swordfish

FALL/WINTER
- Crab
- Scallops
- Oysters

SPRING/SUMMER
- Halibut
- Wild salmon
- Red snapper

Whole Grains

"Whole" means that grains are unrefined and have not been stripped of their bran and germ through the process of milling. Since they are not processed, they are rich in the fiber and nutrients that are present during their natural state. If you see the word *enriched* on breads, pastas, and other grain products, note that some of the lost nutrients (fiber excluded) have been put back into the product—but it's better to just stick with grains that never had them removed in the first place!

Avoid gluten. This isn't a trend or fad, it's the real deal. Your body, my body, everybody's body, does not break down the proteins in gluten easily, so it devours our energy and affects us negatively. Eliminate it from your diet and focus on whole-grain alternatives:

- Quinoa
- Brown rice
- Gluten-free steel cut oats
- Buckwheat
- Whole-grain, non-GMO corn
- Whole rye
- Wild rice
- Sorghum

Oils

When perusing the oil/vinegar aisle for the proper products to incorporate into your homemade dressings and cooked dishes, lean toward the natural oils and steer away from Crisco, butter, or MSG:

- Grapeseed oil
- Sesame oil
- Olive oil
- Coconut oil
- Walnut oil
- Argon oil

Natural Sweeteners

Our country is addicted to sugar. Even worse, we're addicted to the refined stuff that is now the number-one cause of obesity. Now that you're committed to eating clean, you must eliminate high fructose corn syrup, sugar, and sugar's unnatural alternatives (Sweet'n Low, Equal, and so on), and use the real stuff:

- Molasses
- Agave nectar

- Raw honey
- Maple syrup

Legumes

Beans, lentils, and peas are rich in fiber and protein, which helps your digestion and energy. Try cooking with dried beans and pay attention to the difference in texture and flavor. The process is a bit more laborious—you'll have to remember to soak them the night before—but well worth it. If you don't have time for that and need to grab the canned stuff, go for "low-sodium" versions to cut back on your salt intake, and make sure to rinse them well before using.

- Mung beans
- Sprouts
- Lentils
- Garbanzo beans
- Black beans
- Pinto beans

Nuts and Seeds

Aside from the protein these little treats hold, nuts and seeds also contain nutrients that help the immune system and lower inflammation. Stay away from oiled or salted nuts and grab either dry-roasted or raw (you can always roast them at home). Seeds are fun to add to smoothies, yogurt, and salads for a sprinkling of benefits.

- Hemp seed
- Chia seed
- Sesame seed
- Almonds
- Walnuts
- Brazil nuts
- Pine nuts

Essential Dried Spices

- Oregano
- Basil
- Thyme
- Chili powder
- Cumin
- Turmeric
- Peppercorns for fresh cracked pepper
- Sea salt
- Cayenne

Condiments

- Vinegars—balsamic, white wine, red wine, apple cider
- Oils—olive, sesame, grapeseed
- Dijon mustard
- Sriracha or your favorite hot sauce
- Low-sodium soy sauce, tamari sauce, or liquid coconut aminos

Freeze Your Food

I understand that your week can be hectic, and it's nearly impossible to cook and prepare healthy meals for yourself and your family. The freezer is your best friend for saving time and making sure that food doesn't go to waste:

- Herbs

    If you have an excess of fresh herbs, freeze them in an ice tray with either water or broth. Plop them into sauces or other dishes next time you want to add a little flavor.

- Fruits—overripe bananas, berries, pineapple, and so on

    Throw them into smoothies for a creamier texture or use instead of ice cubes in smoothies.

- Artichokes
- Turkey burgers
- Broths
- Soups
- Lean meats and fish

Clean Eating Tips and Tricks

- Don't skimp—eating less than 1,200 calories a day can cause you to burn *less* fat and feel sluggish.
- Eat plenty of lean, high-quality protein from plant and animal sources, including nuts, eggs, and fish.
- Replace refined white-flour products with whole-grain products, including breads, cereals, rice, pasta, and so on.
- Avoid trans fats.
- Eat organic whenever possible.
- Eat free-range meats.
- Eliminate fast food.
- Drink more water.
- Eat every four hours.
- Reduce or eliminate caffeine and alcohol.
- Include a variety of fresh fruits and vegetables every day.
- Cook with olive oil or grapeseed oil.
- Grill, bake, or broil—never fry.
- Avoid canned foods (except tuna and beans). Frozen is fine.
- Eat breakfast.
- Learn to love beans.

If your portions are small, you will want to make sure that you are getting maximum flavor. A small tasty bite is a lot more enjoyable than mounds of food that lack taste and excitement. YogaLean recipes incorporate herbs to enhance flavor, rather than butter and loads of oils.

10

the yogalean one-week jumpstart program and recipes for lean

··

recipes for energy

❧

Pear, Apple, Nuts, and Gorgonzola Salad

Coconut-Almond-Oatmeal-Banana Cookies

Grilled Vegetable Quesadilla

Spicy Chopped Bean Salad

Brown Rice Mushroom Risotto

Gluten-Free Veggie Lo Mein

Chocolate Peanut Butter Banana Smoothie

We can boost our energy in many ways—exercising, drinking coffee, sleeping more, and of course, eating foods that increase it. Protein is a huge energy catalyst and luckily for us, it comes in many different forms—beans, nuts, legumes, seeds, grains, dairy, and animal protein. The recipes in this chapter incorporate a variety of proteins and energy boosters to help maintain long-lasting energy.

When eating animal proteins, our body absorbs the amino acid tyrosine, which helps our brain produce more dopamine and norepinephrine that help with alertness and focus. Meats also contain a lot of B_{12}, which eases insomnia and depression and kick-starts our energy so that it is long-lasting.

Carbs, although often shunned, are a huge source of fuel for the body as they raise levels of serotonin (the chemical that induces good feelings); when consumed via whole grains, they keep our blood sugar and energy stable.

To sustain high levels of energy, ensure that you are incorporating foods with magnesium (found in whole grains and some fish), which converts sugar into energy; fiber (whole grains, beans, fruits, vegetables), which not only helps our digestion but also keeps our energy steady; healthy fats (olive oils, nuts, avocado, fish), as they contain omega-3 that aids in a healthy heart; iron (spinach, chards, kale, red meats), which helps form hemoglobin, the protein that sends oxygen coursing throughout our body.

And finally, stay hydrated. Our body is reliant on water, so make sure you're drinking at least 64 ounces a day and snacking on water-packed foods like apples, celery, pears, and so on.

Pear, Apple, Nuts, and Gorgonzola Salad

SERVES 4

This is my favorite salad! It gives us the healthy fats our body desires, along with a healthy dose of protein to keep us full for a long while. Pine nuts and walnuts are high in iron, which helps regulate the blood circulatory system, and also have a lot of protein—pine nuts have one of the highest protein levels of all nuts. A little note on this recipe—when toasting nuts, the natural oils are extracted, which adds an incredible depth of flavor that enhances the eating experience.

WHAT YOU'LL NEED:

½   CUP WALNUTS, COARSELY CHOPPED
½   CUP PINE NUTS
½   CUP GORGONZOLA CHEESE, CRUMBLED
1   HEAD BIBB LETTUCE, CHOPPED
1   PEAR, SLICED
1   APPLE, SLICED

DRESSING:

2   TABLESPOONS EXTRA-VIRGIN OLIVE OIL
2   TABLESPOONS BALSAMIC VINEGAR
    SALT AND PEPPER

make it lean:

1.   In a skillet over medium-high heat, add walnuts and pine nuts. Toast for 5 minutes, stirring occasionally, being careful not to burn.

2.   In the meantime, mix the dressing ingredients.

3.   In a large bowl, toss the warmed nuts with dressing, cheese, lettuce, pear, and apple.

Coconut-Almond-Oatmeal-Banana Cookies

MAKES 3 DOZEN COOKIES

Coconuts are full of iron, which helps our body avoid fatigue. Mixed with the carbs from the oatmeal, the protein from the almond and oatmeal, and the fiber from the banana, this is a well-balanced energy cookie. To replace the typical oil used in cookies, I recommend coconut oil, which can boost thyroid function and increase metabolism, energy, and endurance.

WHAT YOU'LL NEED:

2	CUPS UNSALTED ROASTED ALMONDS
1	CUP MELTED COCONUT OIL
¾	CUP MAPLE SYRUP
2	LARGE BROWN ORGANIC EGGS
1	TEASPOON VANILLA EXTRACT
1	SMALL RIPE BANANA, MASHED
2-½	CUPS ROLLED OATS, GLUTEN FREE
1	CUP UNSWEETENED COCONUT FLAKES

make it lean:

1. Preheat oven to 350°F. Place almonds in food processor and grind finely; set aside. Using a blender, blend the coconut oil, maple syrup, eggs, and vanilla.

2. In a large mixing bowl, beat the banana, oats, and ground almonds with a mixer. Add the coconut oil mixture and stir until well combined.

3. Drop rounded tablespoons on a nonstick baking sheet.

4. Bake for 12 minutes. Transfer to a cooling rack and sprinkle with the coconut flakes.

Grilled Vegetable Quesadilla

When trying to cut out gluten, look for food alternatives that you are familiar with and enjoy, like corn tortillas instead of flour. Grilling the quesadilla rather than microwaving adds crunch and a smoky flavor. Depending on the season, feel free to swap the veggies and use what's readily fresh and available—zucchini during the summer and steamed butternut squash during the fall and winter. Pay attention to what your farmers are growing and use those as your base veggies. I recommend checking out the Internet for a guide to what's in season when.

WHAT YOU'LL NEED:

1-½	TEASPOONS PAPRIKA
½	TEASPOON GARLIC POWDER
½	TEASPOON DRY OREGANO
½	TEASPOON GROUND CUMIN
¼	TEASPOON KOSHER SALT
¼	TEASPOON FRESHLY GROUND BLACK PEPPER
1	SMALL ONION, CUT INTO ½-INCH-THICK SLICES
1	SMALL ORANGE BELL PEPPER, CUT INTO ½-INCH-THICK WEDGES
¼	CUP SHREDDED ORGANIC MONTEREY JACK CHEESE
4	(6-INCH) CORN TORTILLAS
¼	CUP 2-PERCENT PLAIN GREEK YOGURT
2	SKINLESS, BONELESS CHICKEN BREAST HALVES (ABOUT 4 OUNCES; OPTIONAL PROTEIN)

make it lean:

1. Preheat grill to medium-high heat.

2. Combine paprika, garlic powder, oregano, cumin, salt, and black pepper in a small bowl; set aside.

3. Arrange onion and bell pepper on a grill rack coated with cooking spray. Cook vegetables for 4 minutes on each side or until tender. Remove vegetables from grill and chop coarsely. Lightly sprinkle with dry spice mixture.

4. Sprinkle about 3 tablespoons of the cheese over half of each tortilla; divide

vegetables between the tortillas. Fold each tortilla in half over the filling; coat tortillas lightly with olive oil spray.

5. Heat quesadillas on grill for 2 to 3 minutes on each side or until cheese melts and tortillas are lightly browned.

6. Serve with a dollop of Greek yogurt.

7. If you are using chicken, marinate with the spices for approximately 10 minutes. Grill 6 to 7 minutes on each side.

Spicy Chopped Bean Salad

SERVES 6

With 20 percent of our recommended daily protein intake, these pinto beans and chickpeas will boost your energy and keep you full for a long time because of the fiber. Also, the spice in the chili powder is a metabolism booster. In order to keep it lean, make sure you are either using dried beans (rehydrated via the package instructions) or purchasing the low-sodium canned version.

WHAT YOU'LL NEED:

4	SUNDRIED TOMATOES (PACKED IN OLIVE OIL), RINSED AND MINCED
¾	CUP 2-PERCENT PLAIN GREEK YOGURT
2	TABLESPOONS RED WINE VINEGAR
½	TEASPOON ANCHO CHILI POWDER (OR SMOKED PAPRIKA)
¼	TEASPOON CAYENNE PEPPER
1-½	CUPS COOKED PINTO BEANS, DRAINED AND RINSED
1-¾	CUPS COOKED CHICKPEAS, DRAINED AND RINSED
1	HEAD ROMAINE LETTUCE, FINELY SHREDDED
3	PERSIAN CUCUMBERS, DICED
1	PINT CHERRY TOMATOES, HALVED

make it lean:

1. In a small bowl, mix the sundried tomatoes, yogurt, vinegar, chili powder, and cayenne until well combined. Toss with the pinto beans and chickpeas.

2. Serve on lettuce and top with cucumbers and tomatoes.

Brown Rice Mushroom Risotto

SERVES 4

Risotto is typically made with Arborio rice. Since it is short grain, it holds more starch, which is released in the slow cooking process, giving it that creamy texture that makes risotto so scrumptious. The Mayo Clinic reports that a diet high in fiber lowers cholesterol, improves blood sugar levels, and promotes regular bowel movements. Brown rice contains more fiber than its white counterpart due to the "brown" husk, which not only keeps you full but also gives you energy.

WHAT YOU'LL NEED:

1	TABLESPOON GRAPESEED OIL
1	CUP CHOPPED PORTOBELLO MUSHROOMS
1	CUP SHORT GRAIN BROWN RICE (NOT JASMINE)
2	CLOVES GARLIC, ROUGHLY CHOPPED
¼	CUP WHITE WINE
2-½	CUPS VEGETABLE OR CHICKEN BROTH
⅓	CUP 2-PERCENT PLAIN GREEK YOGURT
¼	CUP GRATED PARMESAN
¼	CUP CHOPPED PARSLEY

make it lean:

1. Preheat oven to 375°F.

2. Heat grapeseed oil in a large oven-proof pot and heat over medium heat. Add portobello mushrooms; cook for 4 to 5 minutes, stirring often.

3. Add rice and garlic; stir to coat well. Add wine and cook until it is almost entirely evaporated, 2 to 4 minutes.

4. Add broth and bring to a boil. Cover the pan and transfer to the oven.

5. Bake for 40 minutes. If the risotto is loose, place it on the stovetop over medium heat and simmer until the liquid is absorbed.

6. Stir in yogurt, parmesan, and parsley. Season with salt and pepper.

Gluten-Free Veggie Lo Mein

SERVES 2

Gluten bogs us down, so it's important to give our body whole grains and nutrients that support rather than hinder. For instance, use brown rice or quinoa pasta, or, if it's fall or winter, use spaghetti squash here. For dishes like this, I love grapeseed oil because it can stand a higher heat than olive oil; as an added benefit, it's an anti-inflammatory, antioxidant, antihistamine, anti-aging, anti-allergic, and much more!

WHAT YOU'LL NEED:

8	OUNCES THIN GLUTEN-FREE SPAGHETTI
1	CUP MUSHROOMS OR VEGETABLE BROTH
2	TABLESPOONS TAMARI SAUCE
2	TEASPOONS HONEY
½	TEASPOON RED PEPPER FLAKES
1	TABLESPOON GRAPESEED OIL
2	CUPS MIXED STIR-FRY VEGETABLES (BROCCOLI, RED PEPPER, SPINACH)
2	CUPS MUNG BEAN SPROUTS (OPTIONAL)
4	CLOVES GARLIC, MINCED
1	TABLESPOON MINCED FRESH GINGER
	PINCH OF KOSHER SALT
1	TABLESPOON TOASTED HEMP SEEDS

make it lean:

1. Bring a pot of water to boil and cook pasta al dente. Drain and set aside.

2. In a bowl, combine the broth, tamari sauce, and honey, whisking to dissolve. Stir in red pepper flakes and set aside.

3. Heat a nonstick wok over high heat and add oil, heating until almost smoking. Add the vegetables and sprouts and cook 2 minutes. Add garlic and ginger and sauté, stirring, for 2 minutes. Toss in pasta, then sprinkle with salt and cook until fully heated.

4. Add broth mixture and simmer, stirring often, for 4 minutes until the sauce has thickened. Finally, transfer to a serving platter and top with toasted hemp seeds.

Chocolate Peanut Butter Banana Smoothie

If you're a peanut butter cup lover, here's your solution to satisfying your cravings. The combination of peanut butter and the protein powder will kick your energy into high gear, and it's great if you're on the go.

WHAT YOU'LL NEED:

½   CUP WATER

½   CUP VANILLA UNSWEETENED ALMOND MILK

1   FROZEN BANANA

¼   CUP ICE

1   SCOOP CHOCOLATE PROTEIN POWDER

2   TEASPOONS UNSWEETENED ORGANIC PEANUT BUTTER

make it lean:

1.   Blend all ingredients until smooth.

recipes for lean

❧

eating for lean is an all-encompassing idea that involves water-based fruits and veggies, fiber, a lot of greens, and a little bit of healthy fat. When thinking about foods that make you feel lean, focus on those that support your digestion, give you energy, and don't make you feel bloated.

For instance, in this section you will see a lot of fiber-enriched foods, such as lentils, black beans, and artichokes, that flush your system and help move things along, clearing your gut and making you regular.

Stock up on veggies; they're low in calories and sugars, especially those like cucumber, which is filled with water, so you can snack on them all day, feel full, and stay hydrated. Other foods with high water content include celery, artichoke, jicama, and zucchini. These will help your digestion and keep you from feeling bloated.

Fruits, although rich in fiber and nutrients, are packed with sugar and will eventually creep up on you and create a foundation that makes you bloated and heavy if you're not careful. However, acidic fruits like grapefruit, which you will find in the Grapefruit and Avocado Salad, help burn fat, and fiber-packed fruits like berries and unpeeled apples are high in vitamins and are great additions to your everyday life.

Before cooking, rinse veggies and fruits, but don't peel them—the peel holds some of the most important minerals and vitamins!

Cucumber Raita

Cucumbers are an ideal addition to achieving YogaLean—their high water content acts as a diuretic and helps eliminate waste products. They're low in calories as well, so it's okay to eat them as a crunchy snack. Incorporating a steady helping of yogurt also promotes healthy digestion because of the presence of probiotics that stabilize the good bacteria in the stomach.

WHAT YOU'LL NEED:

½ CUP GRATED CUCUMBER

1 TEASPOON CUMIN SEEDS

¼ CUP CILANTRO, FINELY CHOPPED

1 CUP 2-PERCENT PLAIN GREEK YOGURT

make it lean:

1. Drain the water from the cucumber by placing it in a towel and gently wringing the excess liquid from it. Set aside.

2. In a skillet, roast the cumin seeds over medium heat for 1 to 2 minutes, stirring occasionally to avoid burning.

3. With a mortar and pestle, grind the seeds into a powder.

4. In a bowl, add the grated cucumber, minced cilantro, and cumin powder to plain yogurt. Add salt to taste.

Lemon Garlic Artichoke Salad

SERVES 4

In one artichoke, we reap lean benefits from its diuretic properties, along with its anti-oxidants, which support a strong immune system, which in turn will help us stay healthy for exercise. Among its abundance of benefits, garlic is a detoxifier that triggers the liver to release toxins from the body—a great aid to maintaining a healthy and lean stomach.

WHAT YOU'LL NEED:

5	TABLESPOONS FRESHLY SQUEEZED LEMON JUICE
¼	CUP OLIVE OIL
½	TEASPOON SEA SALT
1	TEASPOON FRESHLY GROUND BLACK PEPPER
¼	CUP PARSLEY
3	CLOVES GARLIC, DICED
12	BABY ARTICHOKES—FROZEN OR CANNED, CHOPPED
6	CUPS MIXED GREENS

make it lean:

1. In a blender, blend the lemon juice, olive oil, salt, pepper, parsley, and garlic until smooth and thick, approximately 2 to 3 minutes.

2. Toss dressing with artichokes and serve over mixed greens.

Grapefruit and Avocado Salad

Grapefruit is high in enzymes, which burn fats; has high water content; and increases metabolism. The combination of the fruit, cucumber, and lettuce makes this dish bright and crisp, and with the addition of the avocado, you'll have just enough healthy fat to keep your body satisfied.

WHAT YOU'LL NEED:

1	PINK GRAPEFRUIT, SECTIONED
1	HEAD OF ROMAINE LETTUCE, CHOPPED
1	AVOCADO, CUBED
1	ENGLISH CUCUMBER, CUBED
1	PINT CHERRY TOMATOES, HALVED

DRESSING:

2	TABLESPOONS RICE WINE VINEGAR
¼	CUP OLIVE OIL
2	TABLESPOONS FRESHLY SQUEEZED LEMON JUICE
	LOW-SODIUM "SEASONING PACK"

make it lean:

1. In a large bowl, toss the grapefruit, lettuce, avocado, cucumber, and tomatoes.
2. In a separate bowl, whisk dressing ingredients.
3. Toss dressing with salad.

Veggie Soup

When it comes to veggies, we can eat mounds of them without gaining weight; unless, of course, we douse them with Cheez Whiz or oil. Veggie soup is the perfect way to fill up on nutrients, stay full, and stay lean. Also, whoever said eating healthy is bland hasn't flavored with herbs, and this soup is jam-packed with them. But it's very versatile, so if you don't have basil or chives, grab parsley and oregano, or thyme and rosemary!

WHAT YOU'LL NEED:

¼	CUP OLIVE OIL
6	CLOVES GARLIC, MINCED
½	ONION, CHOPPED
½	CUP MINCED CHIVES
¼	CUP CHOPPED FRESH BASIL
	PINCH OF CHILI FLAKES
32	OUNCES LOW-SODIUM VEGETABLE BROTH (OR CHICKEN BROTH)
1	CUP CHOPPED BROCCOLI
1	CUP SLICED MUSHROOMS
1	CUP CHOPPED CARROTS
3	RED POTATOES, CUT INTO CUBES
2-½	CUPS CHOPPED TOMATOES, JUICES INCLUDED

make it lean:

1. In a soup pot, sauté the garlic and onion in olive oil over medium heat for 5 to 6 minutes, stirring occasionally. Add the chives, basil, and chili flakes; stir until combined.

2. Add broth and bring to a boil. Add the broccoli, mushrooms, carrots, potatoes, and any other vegetables (spinach, cauliflower, zucchini, and so on) you enjoy.

3. Lower heat and simmer for 15 minutes.

4. Add tomatoes and simmer for another 5 minutes. Season with salt and pepper to taste.

Huevos Rancheros

SERVES 4

As stated in a 2008 study published in *The International Journal of Obesity*, "The inclusion of eggs in a weight management program may offer a nutritious supplement to enhance weight loss." Eggs for breakfast have been shown to be an important part of a weight management program; when paired with beans, you're giving your body a healthy dose of fiber and protein. Making a traditionally high-calorie meal like Huevos Rancheros lean is easy by substituting high-fat cheese with reduced fat and using Greek yogurt instead of sour cream.

WHAT YOU'LL NEED:

2	TEASPOONS EXTRA-VIRGIN OLIVE OIL
4	LARGE ORGANIC EGGS
4	CORN TORTILLAS
¼	TEASPOON BLACK PEPPER
½	CUP ORGANIC BLACK BEANS, RINSED AND DRAINED
¼	CUP FRESH PICO DE GALLO
¼	CUP FRESH CILANTRO LEAVES
½	CUP SHREDDED REDUCED-FAT 4-CHEESE MEXICAN BLEND
2	TABLESPOONS 2-PERCENT PLAIN GREEK YOGURT
½	RIPE PEELED AVOCADO, CHOPPED
4	LIME WEDGES

make it lean:

1. Heat a large nonstick skillet over medium-high heat. Coat pan with olive oil. Crack eggs into pan. Cover and cook 2 minutes or until whites are set. Place 1 egg in center of each tortilla; sprinkle with pepper.

2. In another pan, heat black beans with pico de gallo and cilantro. Spoon onto each egg and top with cheese, yogurt, and avocado.

3. Garnish with lime.

Lentil Soup

Lentils are an incredible source of protein and fiber, which will help stimulate digestion and prevent constipation and other digestive disorders like irritable bowel syndrome. I like to blend half of the soup to create a comforting smooth texture.

WHAT YOU'LL NEED:

- ½ TABLESPOON CUMIN SEEDS
- 1 TABLESPOON BUTTER
- 1 TABLESPOON OLIVE OIL
- ½ CUP CHOPPED ONION
- 2 CLOVES GARLIC, CRUSHED
- 2 PREPARED PACKAGES OF LENTILS (APPROXIMATELY 4 CUPS COOKED)
- 1 CARTON LOW-SODIUM BROTH (16 OUNCES)

make it lean:

1. In a skillet, toast cumin seeds over medium heat for 1 to 2 minutes, stirring occasionally to avoid burning. With a mortar and pestle, grind the seeds into a powder. Set aside.

2. In a soup pot, heat the butter and olive oil over medium heat. Add onion and garlic; sauté for 5 minutes, stirring occasionally.

3. Add the lentils, broth, and cumin. Bring to a boil, then lower heat to a simmer. Cover for 15 minutes.

4. Spoon half of the soup into a blender. Allow to cool for 10 minutes or so. Blend until smooth, then add back to the soup pot.

5. Heat through, then serve.

Vanilla Berry Smoothie

Berries are high in fiber and water content, which makes you feel full and keeps you regular. This recipe can make a beautiful breakfast or a filling snack—blend it up before you leave for work and pop it in the fridge in the break room at your workplace!

WHAT YOU'LL NEED:

- ½ CUP WATER
- ½ CUP UNSWEETENED VANILLA ALMOND MILK
- 1 CUP FROZEN BERRIES
- 2 SCOOPS VANILLA PROTEIN POWDER
- 1 TEASPOON FLAX OIL
- 1 TABLESPOON CHIA SEEDS

make it lean:

1. In a blender, blend all ingredients until smooth.

recipes for immunity

Beth's Health Salad
Beth's Immunity Soup
Bran Tea
Spiced Carrot Soup with Onions and Garlic
Mung and Quinoa Kitcheree
Moroccan-Spiced Baby Carrots and Beets
Orange Vanilla Smoothie

Yes, an apple a day is good for you, but it also isn't the only thing that will keep you away from the doctor. To ensure that your body is in good health, you need to incorporate a variety of nutrient-enriched foods filled with vitamins and antioxidants and brimming with bacteria-fighting properties.

Produce with beta-carotene, vitamin C, vitamin E, and antioxidants should be consumed to avoid sickness and speed along your recovery.

- Beta-carotene

    Apricots, asparagus, beets, broccoli, cantaloupes, carrots, collard greens, corn, green peppers, kale, mangoes, nectarines, peaches, pink grapefruits, pumpkins, spinach, squash, sweet potatoes, tangerines, tomatoes, turnips, and watermelons

- Vitamin C

  Berries, broccoli, Brussels sprouts, cantaloupes, cauliflowers, grapefruits, honey-dews, kale, kiwis, mangoes, nectarines, oranges, papayas, peppers (red, green, or yellow), snow peas, strawberries, sweet potatoes, and tomatoes

- Vitamin E

  Broccoli, carrots, chard, mangoes, mustard and turnip greens, nuts, papayas, pumpkins, red peppers, spinach, and sunflower seeds

- Antioxidants

  Apples, beans, berries, eggplants, onions, prunes, and tea

An easy way to do this is eat with our eyes—go for color and diversity, because each fruit or vegetable has its own unique nourishing qualities to support our internal organs and health. There's a reason soup is prescribed for the sick, it's because in one pot we can throw in an assortment of veggies to aid in our cure. Also, the heat from the soup, especially if a spicy component is added, will make you sweat, which will help flush out the toxins (if you're stuffy, it will clear out your sinuses).

You will find I use garlic in this chapter, which wards off not only vampires, but also the doctor. With the active ingredient allicin, it will help fight off bacteria and infection. If you're sick, double up on the garlic in your recipes.

Beth's Health Salad

Having a diverse selection of produce on our plate or in our bowl will ensure that we are absorbing the proper nutrients that our body needs to stay healthy. Eating salads with a great amount of veggies will do just that. Red cabbage in particular contains a rainbow of nutrients to keep our immune system at full strength—vitamin C and anthocyanins, fiber, vitamin K, vitamin B_6, potassium, and manganese—and also contains thiamine, riboflavin, folate, calcium, iron, and magnesium!

WHAT YOU'LL NEED:

- ⅓ CUP SLICED HEARTS OF PALM
- ½ CUP COOKED CHICKPEAS, DRAINED AND RINSED
- 4 RADISHES, THINLY SLICED
- ¼ CUP BLACK OLIVES, QUARTERED
- ½ CUP SHREDDED CARROTS
- 1 AVOCADO, CUBED
- 1 PINT CHERRY TOMATOES, HALVED
- 1 CUP SHREDDED RED CABBAGE
- 4 PERSIAN CUCUMBERS, CUBED

DRESSING:

- ¼ CUP OLIVE OIL
- ¼ CUP RED WINE VINEGAR
- ½ LEMON, JUICED

make it lean:

1. Whisk dressing ingredients, then toss with salad ingredients.

Beth's Immunity Soup

SERVES 4

Garlic is an immunity strengthener/saver. It has been called a natural antibiotic because it triggers bacteria and viruses and on its own has high levels of manganese, calcium, vitamin B_1, vitamin B_6, vitamin C, phosphorous, copper, potassium, selenium, and tryptophan.

WHAT YOU'LL NEED:

4 to 6	CUPS VEGETABLE OR CHICKEN BROTH
2	TEASPOONS OLIVE OIL
5	CLOVES GARLIC, CRUSHED
	FINELY MINCED HOT PEPPERS (ADD AS MUCH AS YOU LIKE, DEPENDING ON YOUR HEAT PREFERENCE)
½	TEASPOON CUMIN
¼	CUP CILANTRO
2-½	CUPS CHOPPED TOMATOES, JUICES INCLUDED
	JUICE OF ONE LEMON
	BROWN RICE (OPTIONAL)
	AVOCADO (OPTIONAL)

make it lean:

1. In a stockpot, bring broth to a slow boil.
2. In a skillet, heat olive oil over medium heat. Sauté garlic and hot peppers and a dash of cumin.
3. Add the cilantro, tomatoes, and lemon juice to the broth. Lower to a simmer and mix in the garlic, peppers, and remaining cumin.

OPTIONAL:

1. Add brown rice if you would like carbs.
2. Garnish with avocado.

Bran Tea

SERVES 4

The immunity trinity: honey, lemons, and ginger. A combo of these three helps restore balance to the body's pH, flush toxins from organs and sinuses, provide our immune system with antioxidants, and bolster the lymphatic system.

WHAT YOU'LL NEED:

1	LARGE KNOB OF GINGER ROOT
3	LEMONS
¼	CUP HONEY

make it lean:

1. Cut up fresh ginger root into small pieces; remove rind.
2. Scrub and wash lemons.
3. Boil the ginger root and the skin of 1 lemon with 4 cups of water.
4. Simmer for 20 minutes.
5. Add the juice of all 3 lemons, along with the honey. Stir and allow to cool.
6. Add 2 ounces of brandy, if desired.

Spiced Carrot Soup with Onions and Garlic

The crimson glow of beets is billowing in antibiotics, and the apple a day in this soup will definitely help us feel comforted and healthy. Carrots also have a huge helping of beta-carotene.

WHAT YOU'LL NEED:

1	POUND SMALL RED BEETS, PEELED AND QUARTERED
½	POUND LARGE CARROTS, PEELED AND HALVED LENGTHWISE
2-½	TEASPOONS OLIVE OIL, DIVIDED
¼	TEASPOON SALT
1-½	CUPS APPLE, PEELED AND DICED
¾	CUP CHOPPED YELLOW ONION
½	TEASPOON GARAM MASALA
2	CUPS ORGANIC LOW-SODIUM VEGETABLE BROTH
2	CUPS WATER
1-½	TEASPOONS FRESH LEMON JUICE
¾	CUP 2-PERCENT PLAIN GREEK YOGURT
½	CUP CHOPPED WALNUTS, TOASTED
⅓	CUP BABY WATERCRESS

make it lean:

1. Preheat oven to 425°F. Line a rimmed baking sheet with parchment paper.

2. Place beets and carrots in a bowl. Drizzle with 1-½ teaspoons of oil; sprinkle with salt. Toss. Arrange the vegetables on prepared pan. Bake 40 minutes or until tender, stirring once. Remove from oven; let cool slightly. Cut beets and carrots into 1-inch pieces.

3. Heat a Dutch oven over medium heat. Add the remaining teaspoon of oil; swirl to coat. Add the apple, onion, and garam masala to pan; cook 1-½ minutes. Add the beet mixture, broth, and water; bring to a boil. Reduce heat and simmer for 30 minutes. Remove from heat and let stand 15 minutes.

4.   Place half of the beet mixture in a blender and blend until smooth. Pour blended soup into a bowl and repeat with the remaining soup.

5.   Stir in lemon juice.

6.   Ladle about 1-¼ cups of soup into each of four bowls; top each serving with 3 tablespoons of yogurt, 2 tablespoons of walnuts, and about 1 tablespoon of water-cress.

Mung and Quinoa Kitcheree

SERVES 4

Kitcheree is stew typically made from mung beans and brown rice. I like to use quinoa, however, because it is a complete protein and adds a nice nutty flavor. Because of the spices in the masala, which include turmeric, a spice that helps fight infections, you will feel nourished. For the vegetables, you should pick whatever is fresh and in season.

WHAT YOU'LL NEED:

2-½	CUPS WATER
2	TABLESPOONS OLIVE OIL
1	YELLOW ONION, CHOPPED
½	TABLESPOON FRESHLY GRATED GINGER
1	TEASPOON TURMERIC
1	TEASPOON CUMIN
½	TEASPOON GROUND CORIANDER
½	TEASPOON CRACKED BLACK PEPPER
½	CUP MUNG BEANS, RINSED
3 to 4	CUPS CHOPPED VEGETABLES (CARROTS, CELERY, ZUCCHINI, AND SO ON)
1	CUP QUINOA
½	CUP 2-PERCENT PLAIN GREEK YOGURT, FOR GARNISH

make it lean:

1. In a large pot, bring water to a slow boil.

2. In a large skillet, heat olive oil over medium heat. Add the onion and sauté until translucent, approximately 4 to 5 minutes. Stir in the ginger, turmeric, cumin, coriander, and black pepper; cook for 4 minutes.

3. Add the onion mixture, mung beans, and vegetables to the water; simmer for 10 minutes.

4. Lower heat to low, then add quinoa; cover and simmer for 15 to 20 minutes or until the liquid is absorbed.

5. Serve with a dollop of yogurt.

Moroccan-Spiced Baby Carrots and Beets

SERVES 4

Next time you purchase beets, make sure to keep the green tops, because not only does the root of the vegetable hold an abundance of nutrients, but the greens also contain a plethora of antioxidants and vitamin A, which promote immunity. The bulb itself is full of B-complex vitamins and minerals, including iron, manganese, and magnesium, so with the beta-carotene in the carrots and its natural toxin-flushing properties, this dish will boost your immunity!

WHAT YOU'LL NEED:

1	POUND SMALL RED BEETS, PEELED AND QUARTERED (GREENS RESERVED)
1	BAG ORGANIC BABY CARROTS
2	TABLESPOONS OLIVE OIL
	JUICE OF ONE LEMON
1	TEASPOON GROUND CUMIN
¼	TEASPOON GROUND CINNAMON
¼	TEASPOON NUTMEG
¼	TEASPOON KOSHER SALT
¼	TEASPOON GROUND RED PEPPER
1	TABLESPOON CHOPPED FRESH CILANTRO

make it lean:

1.   Preheat oven to 450°F.

2.   Combine the beets, carrots, olive oil, and lemon juice in a medium bowl; sprinkle with the cumin, cinnamon, nutmeg, salt, and red pepper, tossing to coat.

3.   Arrange carrot mixture in a single layer and roast for 13 to 15 minutes, turning once.

4.   In the meantime, chop the beet greens and steam for 5 minutes or until just wilted. Transfer to serving dish.

5.   Arrange the roasted veggies on top of the greens and sprinkle with cilantro.

Orange Vanilla Smoothie

Oranges, as we know, are full of vitamin C, which helps fight free radicals—or damaged cells that attack healthy cells—that enter our body and cause us to get sick. Adding a vitamin packet to our smoothies too will truly boost our intake of vitamins, especially when sick.

WHAT YOU'LL NEED:

½	CUP WATER
½	CUP UNSWEETENED VANILLA ALMOND MILK
2	ORANGES, SEGMENTED AND FROZEN
2	SCOOPS VANILLA PROTEIN POWDER
1	PACKAGE OF VITAMIN C MIX SUCH AS EMERGEN-C

make it lean:

1. Add all ingredients to a blender and blend until smooth.

recipes for youth

❧

Kelp Noodles

Hummus with Sliced Vegetables

Greek Salad with Roasted Beets, Olives, and Feta

Guacamole and Tomato Salad with Spicy Salsa

Spicy Broccoli Rabe

Salmon Tacos

Youthful Smoothie

Clean eating will help your skin, hair, and nails and support your internal organs to allow you to live longer. Protein-rich foods like beans, eggs, yogurt, and cheese give your hair and nails the nourishment they need to grow and be strong. Protein also provides energy and strength to help your body thrive and even recover when injured or sick.

Probiotics in yogurt not only stimulate a healthy gut but will also benefit our gums and teeth, reducing the risk of disease. Research also shows that whole grains, due to their minerals and vitamins, can protect against diabetes, heart disease, stroke, colon cancer, high blood pressure, and gum disease. This explains why we want to steer away from processed, refined grains—because those disease-fighting components are no longer there!

When piling on veggies and fruits to these anti-aging foods, you will benefit from antioxidants, which combat free radicals, molecules that can cause widespread cell damage and are linked to chronic inflammation, which omega-3s also help to reduce. Also, when you consume a lot of vitamin C, your complexion will become smoother and clearer.

To keep your vision sharp, keep an eye on spinach and other dark leafy greens. These veggies are prime sources of lutein and zeaxanthin, plant pigments that protect our eyes from the harmful effects of ultraviolet light. Leafy greens are also rich in vitamin K, a nutrient that plays a role in reducing bone loss and preventing fractures.

When you eat clean, your body will function better, as it doesn't have to concentrate on filtering out the processed additives, so the vitality of your organs will be sustained.

Kelp Noodles

SERVES 4

Kelp is an excellent source of vitamins and minerals, providing us with 46 minerals, 16 amino acids, and 11 vitamins. When eating for youth, it's important to give skin, hair, nails, and organs a proper dose of all of these things to keep them rich and vivacious. Broccoli, in case you're not aware, improves eye health and the repair of your skin.

WHAT YOU'LL NEED:

8	OUNCES KELP NOODLES
¼	CUP TAMARI
2	TABLESPOONS TOASTED SESAME OIL
1	TABLESPOON AGAVE NECTAR
1	TEASPOON SALT
2	TEASPOONS FRESHLY GROUND BLACK PEPPER
1	TABLESPOON GRAPESEED OIL
2	CUPS THINLY SLICED YELLOW ONION
2	CUPS SHREDDED CARROTS
3	CUPS SLICED SHIITAKE MUSHROOMS
1	TABLESPOON MINCED GARLIC
3	CUPS BABY SPINACH
2	CUPS FINELY CHOPPED BROCCOLI
2	TEASPOONS TOASTED SESAME SEEDS

make it lean:

1. Cook noodles according to package directions. Rinse and cool.

2. In a large bowl, whisk together the tamari, sesame oil, agave, salt, and pepper. Add noodles, coat with sauce, and set aside.

3. In a large sauté pan or wok, heat grapeseed oil over medium-high heat. Add the onion and carrots and cook for 2 minutes, stirring occasionally. Add the mushrooms and garlic and cook for 2 additional minutes, stirring occasionally. Add the spinach and broccoli and cook until spinach is wilted. Remove from heat and allow to cool slightly.

4. Add veggies to noodles and toss until well combined. Garnish with sesame seeds.

Hummus with Sliced Vegetables

SERVES 4

Hummus is usually a combination of garbanzo beans, tahini, and a whole lot of olive oil. Because we're going for ultimate health here, I like to add lentils, which, aside from their energy-boosting properties, also help with hair growth. And lemon? Of course! Lemons detoxify, clear pores, help even out skin tone, and aid in digestion as well.

WHAT YOU'LL NEED:

1	CAN CHICKPEAS, DRAINED AND THOROUGHLY RINSED (ABOUT 15 OUNCES)
1	PREPARED PACKAGE BELUGA LENTILS
½	CUP DICED ONION (OR 1 TEASPOON ONION POWDER)
2 to 3	TABLESPOONS LEMON JUICE
2 to 3	TABLESPOONS LIME JUICE
1	TEASPOON MINCED GARLIC
½	CUP CHOPPED CILANTRO
1	TABLESPOON OLIVE OIL
	DASH OF SALT AND PEPPER
	PINCH OF CURRY, CUMIN, AND PAPRIKA

make it lean:

1.   Toss all ingredients into food processor (or blender) and blend until smooth. If the mixture is too stiff, add water (or tamari for extra zing) until you reach the desired consistency.

2.   Taste and adjust the salt, pepper, and other spices according to your personal preferences. This recipe is very forgiving, full of fiber and protein, and a big hit at a party.

Greek Salad with Roasted Beets, Olives, and Feta

SERVES 4

The Mediterranean diet consists of natural foods and healthy fats. The people who live near the Mediterranean Sea enjoy their meals and take hours to dine, eating slowly and savoring every bite, and it is reflected in the way they look. I love adding celery to my meals due to the crunchy texture, and you can eat as much as you want and never fill up on calories. With its vitamin A, it protects our eyes and prevents aging degeneration of the vision. For the beets in this recipe, it works best if you get a mix of red, candy-striped, and golden beets.

WHAT YOU'LL NEED:

4   MEDIUM BEETS, PEELED AND QUARTERED

4   TABLESPOONS OLIVE OIL, DIVIDED

6   TABLESPOONS RED WINE VINEGAR

¼   CUP FINELY MINCED RED ONION

1   TEASPOON MINCED FRESH RED THAI CHILI OR CRUSHED RED CHILI FLAKES

2   HEARTS OF ROMAINE, HALVED LENGTHWISE AND SLICED ½-INCH THICK AT AN ANGLE

6   CELERY HEARTS, SLICED ¼-INCH THICK AT AN ANGLE

¼   CUP CRUMBLED FETA CHEESE

1   OUNCE NIÇOISE OLIVES PITTED AND HALVED

1   TABLESPOON FRESH OREGANO LEAVES, THINLY SLICED CELERY LEAVES, FOR GARNISH

make it lean:

1. Preheat oven to 325°F.

2. Place beets in a bowl, and drizzle with 1 tablespoon of olive oil. Sprinkle with salt and pepper, then toss.

3. Line a rimmed baking sheet with parchment paper. Assemble beets in single layer on prepared baking sheet and bake for 35 minutes or until tender.

4. Whisk the vinegar, the remaining 3 tablespoons of oil, onion, chili, and a pinch of salt.

5. Arrange beets on 4 serving plates. Drizzle with a little dressing and season with salt and pepper. Top with the hearts of romaine, celery, feta, and olives. Drizzle the remaining dressing all over. Season with salt, pepper, and oregano. Garnish with celery leaves and serve.

Guacamole and Tomato Salad with Spicy Salsa

SERVES 8–10

WHAT YOU'LL NEED:

4   RIPE AVOCADOS, PITTED AND PEELED

3   SMALL TOMATOES, FINELY CHOPPED

1   HANDFUL FLAT-LEAF PARSLEY

1   CLOVE GARLIC, CRUSHED

½   SHALLOT, MINCED

½   LEMON, JUICED

2   TABLESPOONS EXTRA-VIRGIN OLIVE OIL

make it lean:

1. In a mixing bowl, smash the avocados with the back of a fork until you reach your desired chunkiness.

2. Fold in the remaining ingredients.

3. Serve with sliced cucumber, celery, carrots, or your other favorite dipping veggies.

Spicy Broccoli Rabe

Broccoli rabe is the bitter, stockier version of broccoli, and to reduce that bite, we must cook it down a little. Broccoli rabe contains a rich source of glucosinolates, which our body converts to cancer-fighting sulforaphanes and indoles. Studies show that these compounds are particularly effective against stomach, lung, and colon cancers, and promising research hints at protective effects against breast and prostate cancers as well.

WHAT YOU'LL NEED:

8	CUPS WATER
1	POUND BROCCOLI RABE (RAPINI)
1	TABLESPOON OLIVE OIL
1/8	TEASPOON CRUSHED RED PEPPER
3	CLOVES GARLIC, THINLY SLICED
1/4	TEASPOON KOSHER SALT
1/4	TEASPOON FRESHLY GROUND BLACK PEPPER

make it lean:

1. Bring water to a boil in a large saucepan. Cut broccoli rabe into 2-inch pieces.
2. Cook broccoli rabe in boiling water 2 minutes; drain.
3. Heat a large nonstick skillet over medium heat. Add olive oil to pan; swirl to coat. Add the crushed red pepper and garlic to pan; cook 30 seconds, stirring occasionally. Add broccoli rabe to pan; cook 2 minutes. Stir in salt and black pepper.

Salmon Tacos

Salmon is jam-packed with omega-3s and protein, which are key to fortifying your hair and hydrating your scalp. Top it with a cabbage slaw (full of antioxidants, folates, and B-complex vitamins), and you have the taco of youth.

WHAT YOU'LL NEED:

- 1   CUP SHREDDED RED CABBAGE
- 1   CUP SHREDDED WHITE CABBAGE
- 3   CLOVES GARLIC, CRUSHED
- 1   JALAPENO PEPPER, SEEDED AND CHOPPED
- 2   TABLESPOONS FRESH LIME JUICE
- 1   TABLESPOON OLIVE OIL
- 2   FILLETS OF WILD CAUGHT SALMON (ABOUT 5 OUNCES EACH)
- ¼   TEASPOON SALT
- ¼   TEASPOON CRACKED BLACK PEPPER
- 6   CORN TORTILLAS
- ¼   CUP 2-PERCENT PLAIN GREEK YOGURT
- ¼   CUP FRESH CILANTRO LEAVES

make it lean:

1. Preheat broiler.

2. Combine cabbage, garlic, jalapeno, lime juice, and oil in a medium bowl; toss to coat.

3. Heat a large skillet over medium-high heat. Sprinkle fish evenly with salt and black pepper. Coat pan with cooking spray. Add fish to pan; cook 3 minutes, turning fish over once. Transfer to broiler and cook for 1 minute.

4. Working with 1 tortilla at a time, heat directly on the eye of a burner for 15 seconds on each side or until lightly charred. Arrange ⅓ of a salmon fillet in the center of each tortilla.

5. Top each with about ¼ cup of cabbage mixture, a dollop of yogurt, and about 1½ teaspoons of cilantro leaves.

Youthful Smoothie

SERVES 1

Smoothies are great for packing essential veggie/fruit requirements into one cup. Cherries are anti-inflammatories, cancer fighters, sleep aids (containing melatonin—after all, sleep will keep you young), gout preventers, and a perfect aid to manage blood pressure. If you've never used borage oil, run to the store and stock up—it is an anti-inflammatory for the skin, so it will help vitality and hydration all around.

WHAT YOU'LL NEED:

2	CUPS CHOPPED KALE OR SPINACH
6 to 7	FROZEN PITTED CHERRIES
1/4	CUP FROZEN BLUEBERRIES
1/4	FROZEN BANANA
1	TABLESPOON ALMOND BUTTER
1/3	CUP UNSWEETENED ALMOND MILK OR RICE MILK
1	TEASPOON GROUND FLAXSEED
1	TEASPOON BORAGE OIL (OPTIONAL)
1	PACKAGE OF VITAMIN C MIX, SUCH AS EMERGEN-C
1	SCOOP PROTEIN POWDER (HEMP, RICE, OR WHEY)

make it lean:

1. Add all ingredients into a blender and blend until smooth.

recipes for relaxation

Brown Rice and Vegetable Congee

Butternut Squash Soup

Carb-Cutting Zucchini Fettuccini

Sweet Fried "Chicken"

Baked Fall/Winter Fruit

White Chili

Mashed Sweet Potatoes with Yogurt

the key to relaxation is steering yourself away from stress and allowing for a peaceful being. Whether it's a massage, a cup of chamomile tea, or a big bowl of comforting chili, embrace what brings you and your body back to calm.

When stressed, our body reacts—we may experience stomach pain, inflammation, heartburn, and other issues. During this time, incorporate foods that calm your body and bring it back to a normal state, which will then ripple into your emotional well-being.

Foods that have anti-inflammatory components along with fiber, beta-carotene, potassium, and vitamin B_6 help combat the effects of stress and help you relax—foods like olive oil, sweet potatoes, whole-grain oats, veggies, and fruits.

Whole-grain oats help absorb tryptophan, which, as you may know, is the chemical found in turkey that leads to the production of serotonin, the brain chemical that triggers relaxation in the body.

Brown Rice and Vegetable Congee

SERVES 2

Sweet potatoes are high in magnesium, which reduces inflammation. When they are combined with the brown rice and the warm comforting nature of this dish, they will create a calm state with every spoonful.

WHAT YOU'LL NEED:

- 1 TABLESPOON SAFFLOWER OIL
- 3 CLOVES GARLIC, MINCED
- 1 TEASPOON GRATED GINGER
- 1 TABLESPOON SESAME OIL
- 1 TEASPOON MIRIN
- 1 TEASPOON RICE WINE VINEGAR
- 1 CUP BROWN RICE, RINSED
- 2 CUPS WATER (PLUS 1 CUP EXTRA, IF NEEDED)
- 1 TEASPOON GROUND WAKAME FLAKES
- ½ CUP PUMPKIN, DICED
- ½ CUP SWEET POTATOES, DICED
- CILANTRO TO GARNISH
- SESAME SEEDS TO GARNISH

make it lean:

1. In a large pot, heat the safflower oil and sauté the minced garlic and grated ginger.

2. Add the sesame oil, mirin, rice wine vinegar, brown rice, water, and wakame flakes.

3. Bring to a boil, then turn down the heat and allow to simmer for 30 to 40 minutes, without letting the water get too low. Add more water if needed; you want it to have the consistency of a thick soup.

4. Add diced vegetables and simmer for a further 20 minutes or until the sweet potato is soft and the rice is tender. Serve with fresh cilantro and sesame seeds.

Butternut Squash Soup

SERVES 8

Using healthy oils in dishes like this will reduce inflammation caused by stress, and, as you know very well, a bowl of soup will instantly trigger emotional and physical wellness associated with comfort.

WHAT YOU'LL NEED:

- 1 BUTTERNUT SQUASH, PEELED, SEEDED, AND CUT INTO 2-INCH CUBES (ABOUT 2-½ POUNDS)
- 4 TEASPOONS SUNFLOWER OR OLIVE OIL, DIVIDED
- ¾ TEASPOON KOSHER SALT, DIVIDED
- 1 CUP CHOPPED ONION
- 3 CUPS ORGANIC VEGETABLE OR CHICKEN STOCK
- 1 CAN LIGHT COCONUT MILK (ABOUT 14 OUNCES)
  CILANTRO, COCONUT FLAKES, AND SLICED CHILI FOR GARNISH

make it lean:

1. Preheat oven to 450°F.

2. Line a rimmed baking sheet with parchment paper. Place squash in a bowl and drizzle with 3 teaspoons of oil; sprinkle with ¼ teaspoon of salt and toss. Transfer to baking sheet and bake for 35 minutes or until golden and tender.

3. Heat the remaining teaspoon of oil in a large saucepan over medium heat; swirl to coat. Sauté onion till translucent, about 3 minutes. Add the squash mixture and stock. Sprinkle with the remaining ½ teaspoon of salt and bring to a boil. Reduce heat; simmer for 15 minutes, stirring occasionally.

4. Remove from heat; stir in coconut milk. Let stand for 15 minutes.

5. Place half of the squash mixture in a blender and blend until smooth. Pour the blended soup into a bowl. Repeat with the rest of the soup.

6. Divide the soup evenly among eight bowls, and top evenly with cilantro, coconut, and chili slices.

Carb-Cutting Zucchini Fettuccini

Nothing is more relaxing than a plate of warm pasta! Swap out the gluten pasta for rice noodles and faux zucchini noodles, and you will not feel weighed down by the heaviness of the dish. Instead you will feel light and ready to take on the day (or night).

WHAT YOU'LL NEED:

4	OUNCES RICE FETTUCCINI NOODLES
8	MEDIUM ZUCCHINI
2	TABLESPOONS UNSALTED BUTTER
1	TABLESPOON OLIVE OIL
1	CLOVE GARLIC, THINLY SLICED
½	TEASPOON KOSHER SALT
¼	TEASPOON FRESHLY GROUND BLACK PEPPER
½	CUP PARMESAN CHEESE, SHAVED

make it lean:

1. Cook pasta according to package directions; set aside.
2. Slice zucchini thinly to the size of the rice noodles.
3. Steam zucchini until it is the texture of cooked pasta, approximately 2 minutes.
4. In a large skillet, melt butter and heat oil with it over medium heat. Add garlic to pan; cook 1 minute, stirring to avoid burning.
5. Remove garlic from pan with a slotted spoon; set aside in a small bowl. Increase heat to medium-high. Add the noodles, salt, pepper, cheese, and garlic.
6. Toss until cheese is melted and everything is combined.

Sweet Fried "Chicken"

Fried chicken, although dredged in flour, eggs, and sometimes buttermilk, might be one of the most comforting meals our society knows. However, 10 minutes after you're done, the rumbling in your stomach elicits anything but comfort, so I've created an alternative that uses tofu and cuts down the fat and saturated oils to help you remain light and calm.

WHAT YOU'LL NEED:

2	TABLESPOONS RAW HONEY
2	TABLESPOONS BALSAMIC VINEGAR
½	CUP RICE FLOUR
½	CUP WHOLE-GRAIN MEDIUM-GRIND CORNMEAL
½	TEASPOON PAPRIKA
1	TEASPOON GARLIC POWDER
1	TEASPOON SALT
1	PACKAGE FIRM TOFU
¼	CUP DIJON MUSTARD
	OLIVE OIL COOKING SPRAY
4	CUPS STEAMED BROCCOLI

make it lean:

1. Preheat oven to 375°F.
2. In a small bowl, whisk the honey and balsamic vinegar. In a dish, mix the rice flour, cornmeal, spices, and salt.
3. Cut tofu into strips, then dry the tofu with a paper towel or a cloth. Coat the strips with mustard; dredge in flour mixture. Place on a baking sheet coated with cooking spray.
4. Bake for 15 to 20 minutes.
5. Just before serving, drizzle tofu strips with honey mixture.
6. Serve with a side of broccoli.

Baked Fall/Winter Fruit

Apples and pears are both high in fiber and high in water content; this promotes a healthy digestion and makes us feel clean. During the colder seasons, it's easy to devour any baked good and treat in sight, which will leave you feeling gross and bloated. Grab what's fresh, turn your oven on, and warm your house and your digestive fire with this baked goodness.

WHAT YOU'LL NEED:

¼	TEASPOON EACH: CLOVES, CINNAMON, NUTMEG, CARDAMOM
2	APPLES, CORES REMOVED AND QUARTERED
1	PEAR, CORE REMOVED AND QUARTERED
1	TABLESPOON AGAVE SYRUP
1	TEASPOON VANILLA EXTRACT

make it lean:

1. Preheat oven to 400°F.

2. Line baking sheet with parchment paper. Mix the cloves, cinnamon, nutmeg, and cardamom; toss with fruit in a bowl. Add the agave syrup and vanilla and stir to coat the fruit.

3. Place fruit in a single layer on baking sheet; bake for 15 to 20 minutes until very soft.

4. Allow to cool slightly.

White Chili

Sit down and really enjoy a bowl of this chili, taking breaths in between bites and savoring the comfort. With mild green peppers and spices that evoke the Midwest, you can fall into your place at the dinner table and make each spoonful a special moment.

WHAT YOU'LL NEED:

2	TABLESPOONS OLIVE OIL
1	ONION, CHOPPED
1 to 2	TEASPOONS MINCED GARLIC
1-½	CANS VEGETABLE BROTH (ABOUT 21 OUNCES)
2	CANS GREAT NORTHERN BEANS (ABOUT 31 OUNCES)
1	14.5-OUNCE CAN KIDNEY BEANS, LIGHT OR DARK RED
1	CAN CHOPPED GREEN CHILI PEPPERS (ABOUT 4 OUNCES)
2	TABLESPOONS GROUND CUMIN
1	TABLESPOON CHILI POWDER
	CAYENNE PEPPER TO TASTE
1	CONTAINER 2-PERCENT PLAIN GREEK YOGURT (ABOUT 8 OUNCES)
¼	CUP REDUCED-FAT SHREDDED CHEESE

make it lean:

1. Heat the olive oil in a large saucepan over medium heat. Stir in the onion and garlic and cook until softened and translucent, about 3 minutes.

2. Pour in the broth, beans, and green chilis.

3. Add the cumin, chili powder, and cayenne pepper. Increase heat and bring to a boil, then reduce heat and simmer for 10 minutes.

4. Stir in yogurt and simmer for 5 minutes.

5. To serve, ladle into bowls and sprinkle with cheese.

Mashed Sweet Potatoes with Yogurt

If you are in the habit of adding butter and heavy cream to your mashed potatoes, then you should kick that habit—it's not good for you! With the readily available healthy products on the market, it's easy to make substitutes—here you'll get the nuttiness of the almond milk and the creaminess of the Greek yogurt.

WHAT YOU'LL NEED:

4	MEDIUM SWEET POTATOES, UNPEELED AND CUBED
½	CUP UNSWEETENED ALMOND MILK
⅓	CUP 2-PERCENT PLAIN GREEK YOGURT
¼	CUP GRATED PARMESAN

make it lean:

1. Place potatoes in a large pot filled with room temperature water. Bring to a boil and cook for 8 to 10 minutes, or until fork-tender.

2. Drain and place in a large mixing bowl. Add the almond milk and yogurt and mix with a beater until smooth.

3. Fold in parmesan and serve.

metabolism recipes

Matcha Green Tea Latte

Mock Cappuccino with Cinnamon and Nutmeg

Spicy Chopped Salad

Spicy Hummus Wrap

Mocha Smoothie

Spicy Eggs

Spicy Tomato Soup

metabolism is the process that breaks down proteins, carbohydrates, and fat to create the energy your body needs to maintain itself. One of the best methods of increasing your metabolic rate is through regular exercise, but certain foods and supplements also stoke it.

As the Mayo Clinic explains, during the breakdown process, calories in food and drink are combined with oxygen to release the energy our body uses to function. During rest, our body still needs energy for breathing, circulating blood, adjusting hormone levels, and growing and repairing cells. If we aren't consciously assisting the body and balancing out the calorie intake and its ability to burn the calories into energy, then we will gain weight.

The body is an incredible piece of work, as many of its parts function on their own without you even having to think about it. However, in order to sustain longevity, it is your job to support it and motivate its functioning in any way that you can.

A few factors determine individual metabolic rate:

- **GENETICS:** Some of us are born with a high metabolism, meaning that it will work at a higher speed and burn more calories naturally. Those without a genetically speedy metabolism will have to put the time and effort into boosting it.
- **AGE:** At the age of twenty-five or so, our metabolism starts to slow. In fact, it will decrease 5 to 10 percent per decade. Part of this is also due to the fact that when we get older, we become more sedentary. When we were children, our bodies were constantly creating energy by running around the playground, partaking in physical education. Many children can't sit still at all. The other part is that bodies age, muscles decrease, and fat percentage gets higher, regardless of your genetic makeup.
- **BODY SIZE:** The larger you are, the more energy your body needs to move about.
- **GENDER:** Men generally have more muscle and less body fat than women and they use their metabolism a lot more to build on that.

How do you help? Exercise and food go hand in hand when it comes to your metabolism. Exercising will require your body to use more energy, hence it will burn calories to create that energy, and eating will give you those calories to burn. Knowing your body will help you to eat the right amount of calories in order to balance out metabolism and the amount it is burning. That's why starvation doesn't work, because if you don't have calories to burn into energy, your body will store the calories it does have and not create energy.

When planning meals to boost your metabolism, think about your energy and the key components that fuel it: spice and caffeine. Antioxidants are found in a lot of forms and in a lot of foods, but one antioxidant in particular, capsaicin, is particularly helpful when boosting metabolism, as it raises body temperature and releases endorphins. Capsaicin is found in hot peppers. Using these foods and supplements in the proper dosage will assist in achieving

Lean Consciousness. However, overdoing certain stimulants like caffeine- and sugar-laden energy drinks and coffee will burn out the adrenal glands, the endocrine glands that produce and release hormones such as cortisol, estrogen, and testosterone that are essential for functioning. Energy drinks, for one, are filled with sugar and caffeine, which will give you a quick boost of energy and rapidly increase your heart rate but will almost as quickly make you crash. It's important to fuel the body, especially the adrenal glands, so that they can properly give us vitality and energy we need to live.

So let's avoid those foods that make us groggy and tired (sugar, refined carbohydrates, wheat, alcohol) and focus on those that will boost metabolism naturally. Aside from exercising, here are a few tips that will help:

1. Eat smaller meals, but more of them. Eating every three to four hours and including a small protein snack will keep the fires of your metabolism stoked and burning. I like to have an apple and some almonds between meals or a small bit of protein powder with half a banana. A bit of hard cheese and a few carrots are also great snacks.

2. Cut your meal portions in half. If you eat two or three meals a day, consider taking them to half the size you normally would. In thirty days you can train your stomach and mind to want less and be satisfied with less.

3. Add hot peppers—cayenne, jalapeno, and serrano peppers fire up your metabolic system. They will also make your food a lot tastier, and you will naturally eat less as you won't overeat to seek taste and pleasure.

4. Drink more green tea, a drink that is unique in that it has the amino acid theanine to balance out the caffeine and enhance mood; it also provides relaxation to the body. Drinking green tea throughout the day will keep you happy and energized.

5. Add small doses of coffee, caffeine, and matcha—they all increase metabolism. Be moderate—overdoing certain stimulants like caffeine-laden energy drinks and too much coffee will burn out the adrenal glands.

Matcha Green Tea Latte

SERVES 1

Matcha is a form of green tea that is packed full with antioxidants, almost 137 times more than traditional green tea. It also has a healthy dose of caffeine, which is going to fuel your body and get you going.

WHAT YOU'LL NEED:

⅔ CUP HOT WATER

2 TABLESPOONS MATCHA POWDER

1 TEASPOON AGAVE SYRUP

⅓ CUP SOY OR ALMOND MILK, STEAMED

make it lean:

1. Bring water to a boil. Remove from heat and stir in matcha powder and agave until well combined.

2. Pour into your favorite mug and top with steamed soy or almond milk.

3. For extra zing, add a bag of green tea.

Mock Cappuccino with Cinnamon and Nutmeg

SERVES 1

Aside from the caffeine in coffee, which will instantly kick-start metabolism, the dash of cinnamon gives it a nice jolt of flavor!

WHAT YOU'LL NEED:

½	CUP SOY OR ALMOND MILK
	PINCH OF CINNAMON
	PINCH OF NUTMEG (OR, DURING THE HOLIDAYS, PUMPKIN SPICE SEASONING)
1	CUP PREPARED COFFEE

make it lean:

1. Bring milk to a low simmer and add cinnamon and nutmeg. Transfer to a large mug and aggressively whisk until foam is formed.

2. Pour into coffee.

Spicy Chopped Salad

SERVES 1

One of the biggest proponents in boosting metabolism, as discussed, is spice. You can add spice to anything, including your nutrient-enriched salads. Here I add it by tossing peperoncini into the mix and jalapenos into the dressing. In peppers, the spice resides in the white veins, so depending on your heat tolerance, carefully scrape the vein and seeds out prior to chopping, if desired.

WHAT YOU'LL NEED:

½   CUP CHOPPED GREEN PEPPERS

2   TABLESPOONS CHOPPED PEPERONCINI PEPPERS

1   PERSIAN CUCUMBER, CHOPPED

5   BLACK OLIVES, CHOPPED

2   PLUM TOMATOES, CHOPPED

1   CUP SHREDDED RED CABBAGE

⅓   CUP CHICKPEAS

¼   JALAPENO PEPPER, FINELY MINCED (OPTIONAL)

DIJON DRESSING:

½   TABLESPOON DIJON MUSTARD

1   TEASPOON OLIVE OIL

2   TEASPOONS APPLE CIDER VINEGAR

½   CLOVE GARLIC, MINCED

1   TABLESPOON CHOPPED PARSLEY

½   TABLESPOON JALAPENO PEPPER, FINELY MINCED

make it lean:

1.   In a large salad bowl, toss all salad ingredients. Whisk the Dijon dressing mixture in a smaller bowl and then toss with salad.

Spicy Hummus Wrap

Cayenne is made by grinding a variety of dried peppers to form a powder. As with any pepper, cayenne holds capsaicin, which is a key catalyst to your metabolism. If you don't have cayenne, you can use your favorite low-sodium hot sauce or even crushed red peppers for this recipe!

WHAT YOU'LL NEED:

⅓   CUP HUMMUS (SEE PAGE 263)

2   LARGE SWISS CHARD LEAVES

¼   TEASPOON CAYENNE PEPPER

⅓   CUP ALFALFA SPROUTS

½   CUP SHREDDED WHITE CABBAGE

2   PERSIAN CUCUMBERS, CHOPPED

⅓   AVOCADO, CUBED

1   JALAPENO, FINELY CHOPPED

make it lean:

1.   Divide the hummus between the chard leaves and gently spread. Sprinkle the cayenne onto the hummus, then layer the remaining ingredients onto the leaves.

2.   Wrap and enjoy.

Mocha Smoothie

SERVES 1

I love this smoothie because it tastes great and is low in calories and fat, unlike its Starbucks counterpart. Sip it on a warm day and your metabolism will rev up.

WHAT YOU'LL NEED:

- 1 CUP COLD BLACK COFFEE
- 1 SCOOP VANILLA PROTEIN POWDER
- ⅓ CUP UNSWEETENED VANILLA ALMOND MILK
- 2 TABLESPOONS COCOA POWDER

make it lean:

1. Pour the coffee into ice trays and place into the freezer overnight.

2. In a blender, add the coffee ice cubes, protein powder, almond milk, and cocoa powder. Blend until smooth, adding more almond milk, if necessary.

Spicy Eggs

SERVES 1

Eggs, as we learned earlier, are a perfect start to any day. They contain a ton of protein, along with all B vitamins, including vitamin B$_{12}$, which naturally gives you energy. Adding jalapenos (or your favorite pepper or hot sauce) adds that extra kick.

WHAT YOU'LL NEED:

1	TEASPOON OLIVE OIL
1	PLUM TOMATO, CHOPPED
2	CUPS CHOPPED SPINACH
½	JALAPENO, FINELY MINCED
1	WHOLE EGG, 2 EGG WHITES, OR ⅓ CUP OF CRUMBLED TOFU

make it lean:

1.   In a skillet over medium-high heat, add olive oil. Add tomato and sauté until the juices are evaporated, approximately 3 to 4 minutes.

2.   Add spinach and cook 3 to 4 minutes or until liquid is absorbed, stirring occasionally.

3.   In the meantime, whisk the jalapeno and eggs. Add the mixture to the skillet and scramble with the spinach and tomatoes.

Spicy Tomato Soup

With each bite of this soup, your metabolism will instantly feel a jolt. Not only because of heat, which will stimulate your internal organs, but also because of the spice.

WHAT YOU'LL NEED:

1	TABLESPOON OLIVE OIL
1	SMALL YELLOW ONION, CHOPPED
3	CLOVES GARLIC, FINELY MINCED
1 to 2	TEASPOONS CRUSHED RED PEPPER
½	TEASPOON DRIED OREGANO
1	TEASPOON DRIED BASIL
4	CUPS CHOPPED FRESH TOMATOES
2	CUPS VEGETABLE BROTH

make it lean:

1. In a stockpot over medium heat, add the olive oil, onion, and garlic. Stir and cook for 5 minutes.

2. Add the crushed red pepper, oregano, and basil. Stir and sauté for 1 minute.

3. Pour in the tomatoes and broth and bring to a gentle boil. Cover and lower heat and allow to simmer for 20 minutes.

4. Remove from heat and cool for 15 minutes. Pour half into a blender and blend until smooth. Set aside. Blend the remaining half until smooth, then return all of the blended soup to the pot and simmer for another 10 minutes.

ACTION ITEM

Download the YogaLean app to explore even
more healthy recipes.

The YogaLean
One-Week Jumpstart

So you are ready for a shift and perhaps not sure where to start. . . . Let's start with the basics: food and movement. There are many components to the YogaLean program. This jumpstart simply deals with the simplest basics to get you moving in the right direction. Using the jumpstart program, you can clear space to begin your YogaLean program "full throttle" in a week. This eating and exercise program will prime you to desire more positive change in a more serious way. It's never easy to shift old patterns, for they are like worn grooves in the road of life, but it is possible to change, if you apply desire and intention. You may run into challenges this first week, but just remind yourself every day that "it's only a week." Make sure you are doing the affirmation meditation and gratitude lists daily as well.

Meal Plan—Eat This

DAY ONE:

Breakfast: Chocolate Peanut Butter Banana Smoothie (see page 240)
Snack: ½ apple and 5 almonds, 2 cups green tea/hot water mix
Lunch: Salmon Tacos (see page 268)
Snack: ½ apple, 1 cheese stick, and 5 walnuts
Dinner: Lentil Soup (see page 248)

DAY TWO:

Breakfast: Mung and Quinoa Kitcheree (see page 257)
Snack: Green tea and 1 Coconut-Almond-Oatmeal-Banana Cookie (see page 234)
Lunch: Pear, Apple, Nuts, and Gorgonzola Salad (see page 233)

Snack: Youthful Smoothie (see page 269) and 2 cups green tea/hot water mix

Dinner: Veggie Soup (see page 246)

DAY THREE:

Breakfast: Spicy Eggs (see page 286)

Snack: 1 grapefruit and 2 cups green tea/hot water mix

Lunch: Spicy Chopped Salad (see page 283)

Snack: Orange Vanilla Smoothie (see page 259)

Dinner: Cucumber Raita (see page 243)

DAY FOUR:

Breakfast: Grilled Vegetable Quesadilla (see page 235)

Snack: Vanilla Berry Smoothie (see page 249)

Lunch: Spiced Carrot Soup with Onions and Garlic (see page 255)

Snack: 1 Coconut-Almond-Oatmeal-Banana Cookie (see page 234), 5 almonds, and 2 cups green tea/hot water mix

Dinner: White Chili (see page 276)

DAY FIVE:

Breakfast: Huevos Rancheros (see page 247)

Snack: 1 apple, 5 almonds, and 2 cups green tea/hot water mix

Lunch: Greek Salad with Roasted Beets, Olives, and Feta (see page 264)

Snack: Matcha Green Tea Latte (see page 281) and 1 banana

Dinner: Butternut Squash Soup (see page 272)

DAY SIX:

Breakfast: Vanilla Berry Smoothie (see page 249) and 1 orange

Snack: 5 almonds and 1 cheese stick

Lunch: Gluten-Free Veggie Lo Mein (see page 239)

Snack: Mock Cappuccino (see page 282) and 1 apple

Dinner: Spicy Tomato Soup (see page 287)

DAY SEVEN:

> Breakfast: ½ portion Brown Rice Mushroom Risotto (see page 238)
>
> Snack: Matcha Green Tea Latte (see page 281) and 1 apple
>
> Lunch: Lemon Garlic Artichoke Salad (see page 244)
>
> Snack: Green tea, 1 apple, and 10 almonds
>
> Dinner: Beth's Immunity Soup (see page 253)

Exercise Program—Move Like This

> Day One: One-hour walk and YogaLean Energy Sequence
>
> Day Two: 30-minute run/walk and YogaLean Anti-Aging Sequence
>
> Day Three: One-hour walk and YogaLean Anti-Aging Sequence
>
> Day Four: 30-minute walk and YogaLean Relaxation Sequence
>
> Day Five: One-hour walk and YogaLean Immunity Sequence
>
> Day Six: 30-minute run/walk and YogaLean Lean Sequence
>
> Day Seven: One-hour walk and YogaLean Relaxation Sequence

Ten-Minute Affirmation Meditation

Sit comfortably, close your eyes, and repeat the daily phrase over and over again for ten minutes.

You can also do the affirmation during your exercise program and before you go to sleep.

> Day One: I am ready for positive change.
>
> Day Two: Today I am strong.
>
> Day Three: I am peaceful, calm, and relaxed.
>
> Day Four: Today is a new day.
>
> Day Five: I feel good.
>
> Day Six: I have the power.
>
> Day Seven: I am shifting.

Daily Gratitude Practice

Make a list daily of ten things you are grateful for.

Supplements

I love supplements and take them daily. I believe that they keep me balanced, energized, and youthful. If you come to my house you will see a floor-to-ceiling cabinet filled with supplements that benefit my body and give me vitality. The first thing I do every morning is take a handful of pills.

Because of the rigorous processing our food endures, there are a lot of essential vitamins, minerals, and fatty acids that are stripped from our diet but that our bodies require for optimum health. Furthermore, there are certain minerals, amino acids, and other nutrients that are not found in food but are important for our body, especially as we age. Specifically, essential amino acids, which are the components of protein, are not present in food but are incredibly important, because proteins are the building blocks of muscle.

This is why we supplement—to replace lost nutrients, to boost nutrient intake, and to provide our body with nutrients we don't normally digest through eating. Taking supplements regularly will help regulate your body and support its functioning. Vitamin deficiency has an adverse effect on the brain and body, so it's important to ensure we are getting what our body needs in order to maintain itself.

Below are the supplements that I take on a daily basis, which I personalize based on my body and history. It's important to consult a holistic doctor or Ayurvedic specialist before starting your supplementation. This will ensure that you are optimizing your efforts and not taking a supplement that might interfere with medications you are already on or a preexisting condition you have.

Be careful where you get your supplements. The ones you get from a naturopath or health care provider will be of a higher quality.

Basics on an Empty Stomach

AMINO ACIDS

Amino acids work together to build protein. Many are produced naturally in your body, but the "essential amino acids" are found in food sources and through supplementation. In order to reap the full benefits of the workings of protein, it is important to ensure the all twenty of the amino acids are accounted for.

VITAMIN D

One of the most revered vitamins in today's medicine, vitamin D is an anti-inflammatory that helps prevent osteoporosis, treats arthritis, helps maintain a healthy immune system, decreases emotional distress, and can lower risk of cardiovascular disease, diabetes, and certain types of cancer. In its natural form, vitamin D helps stimulate the growth cells in your skin by being exposed to the sun.

L-CARNITINE

Studies have shown that L-carnitine is a powerful ingredient that can help burn fat and aid the post-workout recovery process. It acts as an antioxidant that can inhibit the formation of free radicals, minimize muscle tissue disruption, and promote recovery.

DL-PHENYLALANINE

As one of the essential amino acids, DL-Phenylalanine converts into tyrosine, which produces dopamine and norepinephrine, both of which support the thyroid. This supplement elevates mood, mental energy, sex drive, and motivation. It helps suppress appetite and helps curb cravings. Avoid if you have a history of hyperthyroidism, hypertension, anxiety, or melanoma.

AMLA

A famous supplement known for rejuvenating the skin, amla contains twenty times more vitamin C than an orange. Amla is a vrishya herb, which means that it enhances all the seven tissues (dhatus), including the reproductive tissue, especially in the skin. It restrains pitta, which in turn helps relieve some skin disorders experienced by pitta.

CHLOROPHYLL

As we know, chlorophyll is a green pigment found in plants, which helps plants create food. For us, chlorophyll is a great internal deodorizer that is used to reduce bad breath and oxygenate our blood.

CHROMIUM POLYNICOTINATE

Chromium helps stabilize the effectiveness of insulin, which transports sugar into cells, where it is used for energy. When people who experience problems with insulin, the receptors on the cells do not open and allow the flow of sugar into the cells. Chromium regulates that process and opens the cells.

GINKGO BILOBA

Ginkgo is of great aid to the brain and to blood circulation throughout the body. This supplement is often used to enhance memory and other conditions caused by reduced blood flow to the brain, including Alzheimer's disease, memory loss, headache, vertigo, concentration, and moodiness.

OPTIONAL

DHEA (Women over Thirty-Five)

DHEA is often used by women over thirty-five to regulate the hormones and stimulate human growth hormones. As we age, the production of our hormones slow down, so supplementing for this loss is important. DHEA is also known to decrease cholesterol, boost immunity, and improve cognitive function, libido, and mood by increasing serotonin levels in the brain. Check with your doctor.

Flax Oil and Fish Oil (Omega-3)

They are both popular supplements for body-building and athletic activities; both contain health-boosting properties. Fish oil contains a high amount of the omega-3 acids EPA and DHA. Flaxseed oil from the flax plant is high in another omega-3 acid—alpha-linolenic acid, or ALA, which the body converts to EPA and DHA.

After Lunch or with Meals

MULTIVITAMINS

Taking a multivitamin immediately after eating will help your body absorb the nutrients found in your food as well as add the nutrients that were not present in the meal. A good multivitamin will contain all B vitamins, along with a great many of the other essential vitamins your body needs. If you are a woman, ensure that your multivitamin contains iron in order to make up for the amount lost during the menstrual cycle.

Before Sleep

MAGNESIUM

As we saw earlier, magnesium is an anti-inflammatory that aids in digestion and helps regulate energy levels. Additionally, it is good for regulating both the mood and the bowels.

MELATONIN

Having trouble sleeping? Melatonin will help. It is a hormone produced by the pineal gland, which helps control your sleep/wake cycles. Rather than taking a prescription medication to aid your restlessness, go the natural route.

PRIMROSE

Primrose oil relieves the pain and discomfort associated with PMS, menstruation, menopause, endometriosis, and fibrocystic breasts. The gamma-linolenic acid present in this oil lessens menstrual cramps and may also reduce the premenstrual tenderness of breasts, carbohydrate cravings, and much more.

VITAMIN C

Tests show that vitamin C helps ease upper respiratory infections and reduce bronchial restriction and impaired breathing connected to allergies and asthma. Most important, extra vitamin C improves healthy immune system functioning. It creates healthy blood vessel functioning and helps keep arterial walls clear from blockage, which in turn reduces your risk of heart disease. High levels of vitamin C also suppress your body's release of cortisone, a hormone your body releases during moments of stress. It also prevents bruising.

How to Manage Your Body Type

Ayurveda

There are Ayurvedic daily practices and therapeutic techniques that can encourage a general sense of balance, no matter what your body type is. These tools can help you reduce anxiety, sleep better, feel a greater sense of calm, and detoxify. When we feel a greater sense of overall balance, we can make better choices about food, exercise, and sleep, all of which support Lean Consciousness.

Nose Oils: Nose oils are usually vegetable oil–based (some are ghee-based) and are combined with medicinal or aromatic oils as well as essential oils. You place one to five drops of the oil in the nostril and inhale lightly, both to coat the inside of the nostrils and the sinuses and to stimulate the limbic system of the brain. There are a number of different types of formulas of oils. Some have eucalyptus, and these are more stimulating; others may contain more soothing and calming herbs and scents.

An Oil for Every Mood

After mixing, if the oil smells too strong (for massage), add a base oil that is unscented.

Energy:

Mix eucalyptus and peppermint essential oils.

Calming:

Mix lavender and rosemary.

Immunity:

Mix grapefruit, lemon, and orange.

These are effective tools to support Lean Consciousness because they are traditionally used to reduce anxiety, to calm a racing mind, to help promote sound sleep, and to increase attention and focus. When we are attentive and relaxed, have slept well, and feel clear, we can make better choices about food and exercise.

From an energetic standpoint, the small amount of oil used is effective for calming the erratic, airy vata dosha.

There is a part of our brain known as the limbic system; it includes the amygdala, the hippocampus, and a number of other structures. This is our emotional center, where we process our memories and feelings—everything from joy to anxiety, from happiness to sadness. The olfactory nerves, which connect the nose and the brain, go straight to the olfactory bulbs, which are included within and affect the limbic center of the brain.

Smell has such a powerful effect because the nose is like a superhighway to the brain. Smells carry us back to memories and their associated feeling states, both positive and negative. The pumpkin pie baking in the oven reminds us of Thanksgiving with our grandmother, while chocolate chip cookies might evoke the good feeling we had when we arrived home from school to a warm house. Food is particularly central here since our senses of taste and smell are so intertwined. And when we smell—french fries as we're walking down the street, coffee brewing, or bacon grilling—both our hunger and our memories may be stimulated and need satisfaction.

One of the ways that Ayurveda uses this neural pathway to cultivate balance and support Lean Consciousness is through nose oils.

IMPORTANT AYURVEDIC HERBS

TRIPHALA AND AMLA: Triphala is a mix of three dried and powdered fruits that is one of the most important Ayurvedic detoxifying and rejuvenative formulas. It is said that if all we did was take triphala regularly, we would eventually come into balance. This is important for Lean Consciousness not because it is a laxative type of detoxifier but because it helps the body release what needs to be released at a deep level. Some people find that it dries them out, particularly if they have a great deal of the vata dosha in their body type, so be careful.

Triphala is traditionally taken away from the dinner table (either thirty minutes before or two hours after eating). It has a healing, balancing, and detoxifying effect.

Amla is one of the three ingredients that make up triphala. Any of the three can be taken by themselves, but amla is particularly useful for balancing the hot and fiery energy of the pitta dosha. It is traditionally used for its anti-inflammatory effects, for building muscle, and for healing the skin and the digestive system, connecting it to Lean Consciousness.

TURMERIC: The yellow culinary spice turmeric is one of the most beloved medicinal plants in Ayurveda. While we may know it as the yellow color in mustards and curries, it is increasingly being studied in modern scientific research for its numerous benefits. Turmeric is one of nature's most effective anti-inflammatory agents. Studies have shown it to be even more effective than the over-the-counter and prescription nonsteroidal anti-inflammatory pharmaceutical drugs, without the same side effects. For a person who has inflammation or joint pain such as arthritis, turmeric is traditionally used to help reduce that experience so that a person can exercise much more easily.

Like other anti-inflammatories, turmeric is also good for helping to clear up the skin; it boosts the immune system and has valuable anti-cancer properties. It can also reduce depression. In order to incorporate turmeric in your YogaLean lifestyle, add it (as a diced root or powered spice) to food or smoothies or take it as a supplement. In the Ayurvedic tradition (confirmed by modern research), combining black pepper with turmeric helps to strengthen its effect, so look for supplements that have added black pepper.

ASHWAGANDHA: Traditionally used as a tonic for the adrenals and the nervous system, ashwagandha is a remedy for syndromes related to overwork and depletion. Since an overload of the body's stress response (sympathetic nervous system) has been shown to increase deposits of fat around the abdominal area, addressing the body's stress response through nutritional support is key to maintaining Lean Consciousness.

Some people find that ashwagandha helps them sleep at night, not because it is a sedative but because it has a calming effect on the nervous system. Ashwagandha is a bit of a heating herb; it's good to be careful in the summer or if you have a great deal of internal heat. Ashwagandha is also beloved in Ayurveda for increasing sexual capacity, particularly for men, but for women too.

SHATAVARI: This Ayurvedic medicinal herb is used to strengthen the female reproductive system and balance hormones that can be affected by stress and overwork. In the effort to maintain Lean Consciousness, nutritional support for hormones can be useful to prevent depletion. Shatavari is also used to help reduce the heat and irritation that can occur when the fiery pitta dosha is increased or out of balance.

CHAVYANPRASH: You'll see a number of different spellings of this formula. Often found as a sticky jam, it can be eaten directly off the spoon for a treat that is a combination of sweet and sour flavors. This combination of ghee, honey, and a long list of herbs may not initially seem like a support for Lean Consciousness, but we do need sweet nourishing foods in small amounts. This one is particularly beneficial for its traditional effect on strengthening the immune system and supporting immune health.

11

karma yoga, higher purpose, and giving back

..

One of the best ways to lose weight and gain a better understanding of who we are mentally and physically is by turning the focusing away from ourselves. It's about channeling that energy into a higher purpose through serving our community and world. We all carry a higher purpose in life that is beyond us, and once we connect to that purpose, a renowned happiness will guide us.

Some people get in touch with their purpose with ease, while others struggle to find it. In this section are some ways all of us can find it.

I have had the blessing of being able to see signs from the universe throughout my life. Once in college while I was stretching, I got the profound insight that I would be very successful in the health and fitness industry. On a bike ride in 1994 the name YogaFit came to me. Listening to the universe is profound; it can be an amazing source of guidance and solace—here are some tips to help you in that process.

1. Use introspection to listen to the inner voice that speaks to you during meditation.
2. Learn and understand the difference between a thought and an

insight. We have sixty thousand thoughts a day, and we don't remember most of them. You will know when an insight comes.

3. Understand what in this world touches your heart, whether it's animals, children, seniors, orphans, war veterans, or people with HIV or cancer.

4. Pray to the universe to send you signs and synchronicities.

5. Notice when you wake up with insights and intuition.

6. Journal about your dreams; they can provide powerful answers.

7. Learn to differentiate between a thought and an intuition.

8. Listen for messages from the universe that may come from other people. Like they say in kabbalah—*Look for the signs.* Sometimes people say things "out of nowhere" that are meaningful and can guide you.

Once you've developed an ongoing practice of searching for your higher purpose, you will start feeling and experiencing signs that point you to what that purpose might be. You may also notice that some of your beliefs and practices have shifted slightly, leading you to something greater and more divine. If you are consciously trying to tap into this higher purpose, you will naturally lead yourself to it.

Patricia A. Boyle, PhD, of Rush Alzheimer's Disease Center in Chicago conducted a survey among elderly patients. The study led her to believe that purpose in life reflects the tendency to derive meaning from life's experiences as well as to increase focus and intention.

During the study, which is published in *Psychosomatic Medicine*, she found that a higher purpose in life was associated with a substantially reduced risk of mortality, and the results did not vary according to gender or race. "The finding that purpose in life is related to longevity in older persons suggests that aspects of human flourishing—particularly the tendency to derive meaning from life's experiences and possess a sense of intentionality and goal-directedness—contribute to successful aging," wrote Boyle.

Significant associations with mortality were found with three specific items on the purpose-of-life questionnaire that asked about study participants' agreement with the following statements:

- "I sometimes feel as if I've done all there is to do in life."
- "I used to set goals for myself, but that now seems like a waste of time."
- "My daily activities often seem trivial and unimportant to me."

Continues Boyle: "Although we think that having a sense of purpose in life is important across the lifespan, measurement of purpose in life in older persons in particular may reveal an enduring sense of meaningfulness and intentionality in life that somehow provides a buffer against negative health outcomes."

Finding your purpose is embracing your daily activities or finding ones that make you thrive; setting goals that are achievable; doing more and more to enhance your well-being and keep young at heart; being grateful every day; and most important, giving these things to those around you, especially the less fortunate. No matter your age, there is always something left to give.

Studies have shown that there is a direct relationship among giving back, gratitude, and happiness. How will happiness affect your YogaLean program?

As discussed in previous chapters, you will be more in a flow state when you are happy, and flow states improve your happiness. When we give back, help others, and practice being grateful, our life satisfaction and happiness levels soar.

Why give back? If you have been blessed with the most valuable asset—health—giving back to those less fortunate than you feels like, and is, the right thing to do.

Ultimately, our new YogaLean lifestyle is meant not only for our personal benefit but also the good of those around us. It matters less what we do on our mats than how and why. When we are able to relinquish the desire to be rewarded for our efforts or our actions, then our own good health enables us to give back selflessly to a world starving for more compassion, kindness, and wisdom.

From the Four Paths of Yoga

"Karma yoga focuses on the causes and effects of an individual's actions. It teaches how to live a life of spiritual/right action and selfless service. The true follower of the karma path acts without thought of gain or reward. Karma yoga is a yoga you take inside of you and make a way of life. It is the path chosen primarily by those of an outgoing nature. It purifies the heart by teaching you to act selflessly, without thought of gain or reward. By detaching yourself from the fruits of your actions, you learn to sublimate the ego. To achieve this, it is helpful to keep your mind focused by repeating a mantra while engaged in any activity."

—MASTER VIVEKANANDA, *KARMA YOGA (THE YOGA OF ACTION)*, AN ENGLISH BOOK OF SWAMI VIVEKANANDA, WHO BROUGHT YOGA TO THE UNITED STATES IN 1893

Karma yoga is the basis of the YogaFit company. Every trainee and student is requested to give back, and I urge you to do the same.

I once taught at a spa in Ojai, California, where the women would eat proportioned meals with certain calorie counts and then hop on a treadmill to burn the calories off. I was teaching a yoga class there, and when my session ran five minutes long, everyone would get very agitated. So much rigidity was present. My first thought was that these women have too much time on their hands. Whether we are overeating because we are bored or obsessing over our food intake to an unnatural degree, we need a higher purpose. In his book *Growing the Positive Mind,* Dr. William Larkin states that higher purpose tops the chart of indicators of happiness. At YogaFit we give all our students a higher purpose, starting with our Level 1 training, when we make participants complete eight hours of community service teaching in underserved communities in order to start practicing what they have learned in a traditional class setting.

In order to round out our new practices, we must share what we've learned with the universe, whether it's through projecting our newfound energy and positivity by spending our time with good intentions and giving to those people around us who are less fortunate. When we give, we feel the good of that giving in our minds and body. Watching someone's face light up in response to an act of charity is one of the most joyful gifts we can receive.

There is an extreme satisfaction to donating belongings and time to charity. Studies have shown that philanthropy and the act of giving back go a long way in creating feelings of happiness and personal success. When you de-clutter your kitchen (and beyond) and then donate the goods that are no longer serving you, you permit them to serve someone who is in need.

Charity can manifest itself in many ways, from donating time to donating goods. As an example, cooking for others can be an offering, a means of using your resources to provide for those around you. When wholesome food is prepared and served by hands unconcerned with receiving acknowledgment or praise for the effort or accomplishment, it nourishes the heart as well as the body. Whether you are preparing meals for family, a sick friend, or the homeless, what was once a chore becomes "serving joy."

Ways to Give

Many of these suggestions will benefit others, and doing good for others is karma yoga, and you will reap the benefits tenfold. Recognize the feeling you get and understand that your focus and energy will shift drastically.

1. Volunteer at your local animal shelter or ASPCA to walk orphaned dogs.
2. Volunteer with Meals on Wheels to deliver food to the aged and infirm.
3. Volunteer to read to underprivileged children or the blind.
4. Donate any magazines/books you have already read to senior centers or retirement homes.
5. Donate old towels, sheets, and blankets to your local animal shelter or pet rescue organization. Donate pet toys and food too. Blankets of Love oversees the donation of such items to shelter dogs.
6. Teach a free yoga class to a group of at-risk teens.

7.   Donate body care products to the Visiting Nurse Association or the Nightingale Society.

8.   Donate clothes you have not worn for six months to women's organizations. Donate men's clothes to a shelter.

9.   Always spay and neuter your pets—save lives and stop overpopulation.

10.   Donate eyeglasses to Africa.

A Few Words on Gratitude

One of the most widespread practices in the United States is the conscious act of giving thanks. In *Growing the Positive Mind,* Larkin notes that gratitude is the emotion that produces the most positive reaction in our body. Being thankful, then, literally creates a healthier environment for our mind, body, and spirit. Regardless of what we are bringing with us each day, we "show up" for our lives grateful for the bodies we are living in today and the situations we find ourselves in. Through seeking to accept and appreciate what we have, we find ourselves drawn out of our life circumstances and into our lives. Inevitably, we discover peace and joy.

At YogaFit we incorporate gratitude lists and also the practice of keeping a gratitude journal where on a daily basis you jot down things you are grateful for. In YogaFit's Level 5 training we actually write our gratitude lists after we tear up the list of everything we regret or have remorse for. This can include a belief system that does not serve you. The act of tearing up or burning these lists seems to help us get rid of things we don't need and have been carrying with us. This process should be a regular one for clearing purposes.

Using gratitude lists will help you gain an understanding of what makes you happy and what gives you grace. Your gratitude journal can contain anything you are thankful for—your friendships, summer peaches, the fact that you are able to hold a pose longer than ever before, or simply the sun. As with any journal, there should be no judgment when penning your thanks. Start with three items a day.

May we be always grateful for many things, in many ways—always.

Namaste.

appendix a

Vata

Characteristics of Vata

Vata is composed of the elements of air and ether (empty space); it is often known simply as the air element. The predominant characteristics of vata are that it is light, dry, cold, expansive, rough, movable, changeable, and erratic.

The vata dosha controls the overall movement in the body, including speech and hearing, the movement of impulses through the nervous system, and the movement of the musculature of the digestive system (peristalsis).

Physical: the classic ectomorph: slender, with light, often birdlike bone structure and sometimes with prominent, bony, or cracking joints. There is often a tendency toward dryness throughout the body, including in the hair, nails, skin, joints, and digestive system.

These thin, slender people can actually find it challenging to gain weight or to build muscle. (But this doesn't mean that they are automatically gifted with the true nature of Lean Consciousness or that they are, by default, YogaLean.)

Mental/Emotional: quick-moving thoughts, strong intuition and insight, jumping from one thing to another, the ability to connect the dots and use creativity strongly. Sometimes they can be flighty, easily distracted, anxious, and fearful.

NEGATIVES OF THIS BODY TYPE

Physical: Vatas have a tendency toward anxiety and with this comes physical complications such as dry or cracked skin, constipation, premature wrinkles, creaky joints, gassiness and bloating, overly fast digestion of food, alternating constipation and diarrhea, low digestive strength or fire, increased risk of osteoporosis, and cold hands and feet.

Even a person with an abundance of the vata dosha can end up out of balance and gain weight. If you've ever felt "skinny fat," lacking muscle tone, this is an example of what it can look like when vata is out of balance.

Mental/Emotional: Some of the pitfalls of this body type relate to emptiness and spaciness: irregularity both mentally and physically, including fearfulness, feelings of being ungrounded, forgetfulness, emptiness, depression, anxiety, worry, always losing keys or locking yourself out of the house, ringing in the ears, restless leg syndrome, jitteriness, lack of ability to pay attention, mind racing, and more.

Food: When vata energy is out of balance, and a person feels overwhelmingly empty or anxiety-ridden, a person may try to reduce the anxiety and fill themselves in any way possible—including overeating. Since the vata digestion tends to be irregular, overeating is particularly harmful, as the body may not fully digest the food and nutrients. Cravings can set in, and a person may continue to eat trying to feel full or satisfied.

Vata-predominant people will be the most likely to skip meals, either because they love feeling empty, they are not hungry, or they don't want to be bothered with food (it's too much trouble, or they just forgot). Not eating consistently or regularly can interfere with your metabolism as well as your digestive or metabolic fire. While you may want to stop eating in order to obtain the body you desire, throwing off the metabolic pendulum by skipping meals, restricting calories below what is healthy, engaging in irregular habits and schedules, or under-nourishing yourself will work against you when it comes to Lean Consciousness. Additionally, irregular digestion can also interfere with the ability to maintain a state of Lean Consciousness.

In order to maintain balance, regular mealtimes; small, frequent meals; warm and cooked foods; and having snacks on hand are all important.

Sleep: Just as digestion can be irregular, so is sleep. It's the vata-predominant or out-of-balance person who has trouble either falling asleep or staying asleep (often waking up between 2 and 4 A.M.). Since sleep is an important regulator of our body's ability to maintain healthy, appropriate, and lean weight, a vata person whose sleep patterns are thrown off will have more trouble maintaining a healthy, lean weight.

Encourage sound sleep with soothing herbs like ashwagandha, chamomile tea, warm almond or dairy milk before bed, or a gentle foot massage at night. A simple meditation practice that can be done even while beneath the sheets can help calm your often-racing mind.

Patterns of Weight Gain: If you've caught yourself whispering "thunder thighs" to yourself while looking at the mirror, you feel a sense of despair at the way your skinny jeans just don't fit, or if your weight gain is disproportionately in your lower body (hips and thighs), this reveals a vata imbalance. The classic vata weight imbalance is the pear shape, or weight gain in the hips, thighs, glutes, and lower body.

POSITIVES OF THIS BODY TYPE

Vata, being the dosha or the body type of movement, lightness, and creativity, has many gifts and positive qualities. People with strong vata posses a sense of excitement and adventure. You're always willing to pack your bag and take off (even if you might lose your house keys along the way). You love stimulation and are always chasing the new and the novel. The expansive vata-type mind is creative, full of curiosity, intuitive, insightful, and often even psychic.

Vatas love movement, but since stamina isn't always their strong suit, it is important to work up to intense workouts and not burn out with enthusiasm all in one day. This love of movement can manifest as its best self with gracefulness and ease.

Pitta

Characteristics of Pitta

A mesomorph, or person in the middle, matches up with the Ayurvedic dosha pitta. While pitta represents the element of fire, it is neither as light as vata nor as heavy as kapha. People who have a strong pitta body type are often of medium build with a medium bone structure. Good news for gym-lovers: The person with a predominant pitta dosha has the easiest time building muscle.

Physical: The pitta dosha (fire element) governs all digestion and metabolism. This is not merely limited to the digestive system but includes digestion within the cells and the tissues, detoxification and other metabolic processes that take place in the liver, and the digestion and assimilation of the experiences that take place in the mind.

Because there is so much internal fire, people with this body type do not like to skip a meal, and may even wake up hungry. If you are a person with this body type or live with one, carry snacks to maintain blood sugar and the appropriate conditions for metabolic consistency.

This presence of fire can be seen in many of the physical and mental characteristics of the pitta body type. They may have red or ruddy skin that burns easily or have a tendency toward rosacea, inflammation, or irritation. You may see the fire in their eyes (or your own). People with a strong pitta body type may even possess a radiance that shines from their eyes and their entire bodies. There is a bit of oiliness in the body of people with this type.

Mental/Emotional: The energetic fire also relates to desire, excitement, discernment, judgment, discipline, competition, and our ability to dive right into a project or passion as well as the ability to chase our dreams and the ability to manifest. This also relates to the process of transformation. Since people with the pitta body type have a high degree of natural competition, the important thing is not to completely suppress it but rather to develop a healthy relationship with competition, one that pushes you toward excellence.

NEGATIVES OF THIS BODY TYPE

Physical: One of the challenges of this body type from an Ayurvedic perspective is the tendency toward inflammation and the sensitivity to sugar, caffeine, and other stimulants. One of the dangers of the apple-shaped imbalance, or the creeping waistline, is that it is linked to a greater risk of heart attack in both men and women. There is also a danger here that the internal fire can burn your own tissues, increasing the risk of any imbalances that are heat-related, such as inflammation, ulcerations, high blood pressure, and skin disorders.

Mental/Emotional: The person with a pitta-predominant constitution or who is manifesting a pitta imbalance is the classic Type A personality. This is the person (it may even be you) who weaves around traffic, is friendly with the car horn, can crank out a nasty email in five seconds flat, and lives life on the adrenaline high of the constant roller coaster ride.

From a mental/emotional standpoint, the challenge of the pitta dosha is the imbalance of the fire element. These people, when angry, can destroy everything in their path.

Food: While any body type or tendency can fall prey to stress eating, the pitta type is particularly susceptible, coupled with an increased risk of heart disease, high blood pressure, and weight around the belly is often created by excess cortisol. Caffeine can drive up blood sugar and be a further complicating factor, along with the intense hunger that can accompany stress. A regular schedule of workouts and eating meals at a consistent time are both important. (Skipping meals can trash both your mood as well as your ability to make good choices about food.)

Sleep: It's the person with a predominance or imbalance of this tendency who may have trouble falling asleep. Why would you want to sleep when there's already so much on the to-do list or when it has been a demanding day and there's a lot of planning going on? Or you may feel an overwhelming hunger late at night, and that big meal is making it hard to fall asleep. The drawback to this is that a good night of sleep helps to balance and coordinate the hormone cascade that controls hunger; our body produces growth hormone in those early hours of sleep, allowing us to repair and build healthy muscle tissue. Even though falling asleep at night may be a challenge, employing techniques such as a meditation or stress reduction practice at night, warm milk or herbal tea before bed, or a YogaFit workout regimen that promotes sound sleep are crucial for balance.

Patterns of Weight Gain: While the medium build, medium stamina, and desire for excellence are ingredients for a recipe for Lean Consciousness, the pitta body type must beware of the accumulation of the stress response. The weight gain pattern of pitta out of balance is the apple from the fruit bowl. This is also related to abdominal fat deposition as a result of cortisol buildup.

POSITIVES OF THIS BODY TYPE

The medium frame and natural intensity of the pitta-predominant body type creates the ability to develop Lean Consciousness easily—with the right amount of dedication. Discipline is one of the natural positive qualities of this tendency and can be put to good use physically through working out, sticking to a particular eating program, and incorporating a regular meditation practice. The drive and passion of the pitta body type, when directed appropriately, can give a person a sense of drive and purpose. The pittas are the go-getters. The positive qualities of the Type A or passionate personality of getting things done, incorporating qualities of discernment to make good decisions, and building healthy muscular strength are well developed. Physically, pitta-type people are well-proportioned when lean.

Kapha

Characteristics of Kapha

The endomorph is characteristic of the kapha-predominant type of person. These are the people who can both build structure and hold on to weight, fluid, and substance. The challenge here is to utilize the innate strength of the physical body without becoming stagnant.

Physical: Something to note here is that even the healthiest of this body type is not going to look lean like a vata person will. The combination of dense bone structure, natural insulation, and heavy muscle will give this type a different look of lean.

They may not naturally buy themselves a gym membership for a gift, but these are the people who have the most stamina and need to incorporate the strongest types of physical activity in their daily routine in order to maintain balance and cultivate Lean Consciousness.

Mental/Emotional: The kapha dosha is connected to unconditional love, familial love, long-term memory, steadiness and commitment, and security and safety, with a strong tendency to follow through to completion. This body type possesses persistence and the ability to see a project through to the end and also has the quality of being a sustainer.

The kapha body type is a homemaker, a cook, a person who excels at nourishing themselves and others. While a vata type might skip a meal because they forgot, a kapha person will never miss the opportunity for a meal if they can help it.

NEGATIVES OF THIS BODY TYPE

Physical: Since the kapha type often has a tendency for a naturally voluptuous, soft body, the danger is that when it is out of balance, instead of being strong and muscular, the stagnation can lead to a physical form that is closer to the Pillsbury Doughboy than an Olympic swimmer or power lifter. This body type can end up heavy, weighed down, stuck, stagnant, or soggy. There can be a tendency toward being overweight, or even developing growths or tumors. Sluggishness can take hold anywhere, including in the digestive system, in circulation, in the skin, and in the metabolism as a whole. The person with a predominance of the kapha dosha needs to be heated up and worked out. Sweating every day and eating warm spicy foods are essential to keep stagnation from taking hold.

Mental/Emotional: Just as the kapha body can end up being stuck, so can the kapha mind. This tendency can lead to an increase in stubbornness, resistance to change, an inability to see anything other than his or her own point of view, and an attachment to comfort. Sometimes it takes a lot of effort for people with this strong tendency to change their routine.

Food: People with a strong kapha tendency can have a little too much love of comfort foods and sweets. They love to cook and seldom miss the opportunity to enjoy a meal or a snack. The danger is that these heavy foods can further increase their natural heaviness. Hot water with lemon, raw foods (especially vegetables), light snacks, and small meals are all important practices that help reduce this tendency for imbalance.

Sleep: This type has a tendency toward stability. The challenge here isn't falling asleep but sleeping too much or having trouble waking up in the morning with a bounce in your step. While we know that we need sleep in order to maintain Lean Consciousness, it is possible to have too much of a good thing. Try getting up earlier than usual, set the coffee pot the night before, set up morning appointments with a workout buddy so that there is accountability for the morning sweat, hire a trainer, look for the neighborhood's sunrise YogaFit classes, consider biking or walking to work.

Patterns of Weight Gain: The classic area of weight gain related to the energetic quality of Kapha is the upper chest, shoulders, back, and upper arms. Proportionally greater weight gain here, or generalized obesity—these are signatures of this body tendency pattern of weight gain.

POSITIVES OF THIS BODY TYPE

The healthy, beautiful version of this type is a person with a great deal of stamina, a well-developed chest (muscular or well-endowed), soft and thick skin, and the ability to sleep well and remember forever.

CHAKRA CHART

Seventh Chakra—CROWN
Located at the top of the head
Affirmation: "I Am," "I Understand"
Spiritual center, development of psychic abilities, enlightenment, unity
Balancing this chakra helps the central nervous system, muscular system, skin

Sixth Chakra—THIRD EYE

Located in the center of the forehead

Affirmation: "I Know," "I Think"

Perception center, psychic consciousness, wisdom, intuitive ability, visualization, power of mind

Balancing this chakra helps the brain and nervous system, eyes, ears, nose

Fifth Chakra—THROAT

Located in the center of the throat

Affirmation: "I Speak," "I Express"

Expression center, communication, inner voice, speaking from truth, expression of creativity (arts, music), willpower

Balancing this chakra helps the throat and thyroid, esophagus, trachea, mouth, jaw, teeth, neck, vertebrae

Fourth Chakra—HEART

Located in the center of the chest

Affirmation: "I Love"

Love center, compassion, unconditional love, hope, forgiveness

Balancing this chakra helps the heart, circulatory system, ribs, breast, thymus gland, lungs, shoulders, arms, hands, diaphragm

Third Chakra—SOLAR PLEXUS

Located in the area above the navel

Affirmation: "I Can," "I Do"

Power center, self-confidence and esteem, manifestation

Balancing this chakra helps the stomach, pancreas, adrenals, upper intestines, liver, gall bladder, middle spine

Second Chakra—SACRAL

Located in the lower abdomen, genitals, womb

Affirmation: "I Feel," "I Want"

Creativity and sexuality; relationship with money, career, and power; procreation; ability to feel joy and pleasure.

Balancing this chakra helps the sexual organs, large intestine, lower vertebrae, pelvis, hip area, urinary bladder

First Chakra—ROOT

Located at the base of the spine

Affirmation: "I Do," "I Am"

Survival and security center, family connections, animal instinct, controls fear, helps in grounding

Balancing this chakra helps the spinal column, rectum, legs, bones, feet. Energizes body, increases overall health

appendix b

Techniques
(What Are They and
How Do They Work?)

Ayurveda and yoga include techniques to increase the digestive fire and improve elimination. When our digestive systems are working effectively and efficiently, then we eat just the right amount of food to nourish ourselves and maintain our health and well-being.

Practices that strengthen the digestive organs and abdominal musculature also help us improve our posture, maintain a lean silhouette, reduce bloating and discomfort, and support proper elimination.

Abdominal Lift: The first part of any of these, and a strong practice in and of itself, the abdominal lift starts to train the abdominal muscles and supports tone in the digestive system.

One way that we can do this is sideways in front of a mirror to observe the full effect.

While standing with knees bent, inhale deeply, then exhale fully and lean slightly forward. With the breath held out, draw the abdominal muscles in and up from the lowest part of the abdominal area (between the navel and pubic bone) as far as you can. Continue to pull the muscles in gently as long as you can maintain the breath held out. When you are ready to breathe, relax the muscles first.

Nauli: This is a bit of a yoga party trick pose. It doesn't really matter whether or not you get the pose "right." Just the process of practicing it has a beneficial effect that is the next level of progression beyond the first two techniques.

For nauli, begin in the same way as the first practice. After you have exhaled fully and drawn in the abdominal muscles, then relax them and pull in on the obliques one side at a time. The obliques are the diagonal muscles on the sides of the torso. As you pull in on the obliques on one side, and you allow the rectus abdominis, or the center of the abdominal muscles, to push forward, you will then rotate the center of the abdominals, the rectus abdominis, in circles, creating a churning action. You can move in one direction only, or you can alternate circular directions. When you are ready to breathe, relax everything first and then inhale deeply.

This churning action further deepens the purifying, fire-stimulating, and abdominal toning effects of these practices.

acknowledgments

t o start, run, and grow a business, even a yoga business, is not an easy task. It requires commitment, persistence, and dedication.

I thank the universe for the opportunity to transform continually and to evolve myself to keep the network moving forward.

This book is dedicated to the YogaFit Network and family. If not for your love, support, encouragement, and presence, I would not be inspired to keep moving forward on my own path.

I'd like to acknowledge YogaFit's Master Trainers, who go out into the field every weekend and facilitate growth, inspiration, and transformation, using yoga as the gateway to a healthier life.

A special acknowledgment to my partner, Esra, for giving me amazing love, support, and the opportunity to finally achieve work/life balance.

Big thanks to Danielle Bernabe for helping crystallize my thoughts and tangents into structure; Will Hobbs for his warlike strategy and road map; my editor, Marnie Cochran, for having patience with my Siri Mania; Jenny Baldwin for combing through content while running YogaFit's monthly Mind Body Fitness Conferences; Sandi Cartwright Call for her loyalty to YogaFit since 1998; Heidi Dix for spearheading YogaFit's 1000 Hour Yoga Therapy Program to success; Tracy Jennings Hill for bringing YogaFit groups to India every year; Felicia Tomasko for Ayurvedic inspiration; Shaye Moledyke for creating YogaFit Warriors Program; Lisa Greenbaum for keeping Canada humming; Dr. Pam Peeke for turning me on to Transcendental Meditation; Dr. Lorene Hiris of the Post Campus of Long Island University for guidance and advice for over twenty years.

A special shout-out to my friends who knew me before any of this "Yoga" happened.

And of course . . . my dog, Bentley, for constant canine companionship.

bibliography

ACE Lifestyle and Weight Management Consultant Manual: Second Edition. ACE, 2008.

Akers, Brian Dana (trans.). *The Hatha Yoga Pradipika: The Original Sanskrit, Svatmarama.* YogaVidya, 2002.

Amen, Daniel G. *Change Your Brain, Change Your Body: Use Your Brain to Get and Keep the Body You Have Always Wanted.* New York: Three Rivers, 2010.

Benagh, Barbara. "How Healthy Is Your Breathing?" *Yoga Journal* (March 15, 2011). www.yogajournal.com/practice/218.

Bennett, Drake. "Eat Popcorn, Be Immune to Advertising." *Bloomberg BusinessWeek*, October 14, 2013. www.businessweek.com/articles/2013-10-14/eat-popcorn-be-immune-to-advertising.

Coelho, Paulo. *The Alchemist.* New York: HarperCollins Publishers, 1993.

Cotton, Richard T., and Ross E. Andersen. *ACE Clinical Exercise Specialist Manual.* ACE, 1999.

Csikszentmihalyi, Mihaly. *Flow: The Psychology of Optimal Experience.* New York: Harper & Row, 1990.

Dale, Cyndi, and Richard Wehrman. *The Subtle Body: An Encyclopedia of Your Energetic Anatomy.* Boulder, CO: Sounds True, 2009.

Das, Lama Surya. *Words of Wisdom.* Hawaii: Koa Books, 2008.

Easwaran, Eknath. *Essence of the Upanishads: A Key to Indian Spirituality.* Tomolas, CA: Nilgiri Press / Blue Mountain Center for Meditation, 1981, 2009.

Fain, Jean. *The Self-Compassion Diet: A Step-by-Step Program to Lose Weight with Loving-Kindness.* Boulder, CO: Sounds True, 2011.

Farhi, Donna. *Bringing Yoga to Life.* New York: HarperCollins, 2005.

Feldman, Christina. *Beginner's Guide to Buddhist Meditation.* California: Rodmell Press, 2006.

Feuerstein, Georg. *The Yoga Tradition.* Prescott, AZ: Hohm, 1998.

Gage, Randy. "Achieving Self-Mastery." Get Motivation (nd) getmotivation.com/articlelib/articles/rgage_selfmast.html

Griffith, H. Winter. *Minerals, Supplements, & Vitamins: The Essential Guide.* Arizona: Fischer Books LLC, 2000.

Hanh, Thich Nhat, and Nguyen Anh-Huong. *Walking Meditation.* Boulder, CO: Sounds True, 2006.

Iyengar, B. K. S. *Light on Pranayama: The Yogic Art of Breathing.* New York: Crossroad, 1988.

Iyengar, B. K. S. *Light on Yoga: Yoga Dipika.* London: Unwin Paperbacks, 1968.

Knapp, Caroline. *Appetites: Why Women Want.* New York: Counterpoint, 2003.

Larkin, William Kent. *Growing the Positive Mind with the Emotional Gym and the Positive Mind Test*. Rancho Mirage: Applied Neuroscience, 2008.

Lee, Al, and Don Campbell. *Perfect Breathing*. New York: Sterling Publishing, 2009.

Magner, Marcia Zina. *31 Words to Create an Organized Life*. Hawaii: Inner Ocean Publishing, 2006.

Marrone, Margo. *The Organic Pharmacy*. New York: Duncan Baird Publishers, 2009.

Mayo Clinic. "Nutrition and Healthy Eating." Mayo Foundation for Medical Education and Research (n.d.) www.mayoclinic.com/health/organic-food/NU00255/NSECTIONGROUP=2

Mayo Clinic. "Whole Grains: Hearty Options for a Healthy Diet." Mayo Foundation for Medical Education and Research (n.d.) www.mayoclinic.com/health/whole-grains/NU00204

Michaels, Jillian, and Mariska Van Aalst. *Master Your Metabolism: The 3 Diet Secrets to Naturally Balancing Your Hormones for a Hot and Healthy Body!* New York: Crown, 2010.

Mitchell, Stephen. *Bhagavad Gita: A New Translation*. New York: Harmony Books, 2000.

"Nutrition Coaching." iChange (Fall 2010). www.ichange.com.

Palmer, Brooks. *Clutter Busting Your Life: Clearing Physical and Emotional Clutter to Reconnect with Yourself and Others*. California: New World Library, 2012.

Patañjali, J. R., S. B. Tailang Ballantyne, and Govind Sastri Deva. *Yoga Sutras*. Delhi: Parimal Publications, 1983.

Peake, Pam, MD, MPH, FACP. *Hunger Fix*. New York: Rodale, 2012.

Radhakrishnan, S. *The Principal Upanishads*. New York: Harper, 1953.

Ricard, Matthieu. *Happiness: A Guide to Developing Life's Most Important Skill*. New York: Little, Brown and Company, 2006.

Rosen, Richard, and Kim Fraley. *The Yoga of Breath: A Step-by-Step Guide to Pranayama*. Boston: Shambhala, 2002.

Roth, Geneen. *When Food Is Love: Exploring the Relationship between Eating and Intimacy*. New York: Dutton, 1991.

Roth, Geneen. *Women, Food and God: An Unexpected Path to Almost Everything*. New York: Scribner, 2010.

Rush University Medical Center. "Having a Higher Purpose in Life Reduces Risk of Death Among Older Adults." (June 12, 2009). www.rush.edu/webapps/MEDREL/servlet/NewsRelease?ID=1232

Saradananda, Swami. *Chakra Meditation: Discover Energy, Creativity, Focus, Love, Communication, Wisdom, and Spirit*. London: Duncan Baird Publishers, 2008.

Shapiro, Debbie. *Your Body Speaks Your Mind: How Your Thoughts and Emotions Affect Your Health*. Freedom, CA: Crossing, 1997.

Shaw, Beth. *Beth Shaw's YogaFit*. Champaign, IL: Human Kinetics, 2009.

Shaw, Beth. YogaFit® YogaLean™ Training Manual Level I, 2011.

Shaw, Beth. YogaFit® YogaLean™ Training Manual Level II, 2011.

Shaw, Beth. YogaFit® Level 2 Training Manual, 2013.

Shaw, Beth. YogaFit® Pranayama Training Manual, 2011.

Siff, Jason. *Unlearning Meditation: What to Do When the Instructions Get in the Way*. Boston: Shambhala. 2010.

Sparrowe, Linda, and Patricia Walden. *The Woman's Book of Yoga and Health: A Lifelong Guide to Wellness*. Boston: Shambhala, 2002.

Spurlock, Morgan (director). *Supersize Me*. Produced by The Con and Kathbur Pictures, in association with Studio on Hudson, 2004.

Stanway, Penny. *The Miracle of Lemons: Practical Tips for Health, Home, and Beauty*. London: Watkins Publishing, 1988.

Svātmārāma, Swami, and Pancham Sing. *The Hatha Yoga Pradipika*. New York: AMS, 1974.

Tolle, Eckhart. *The Power of Now*. California: New World Library, 2004.

Vasu, Śrīśa Chandra. *The Gheranda Samhita*. New Delhi: Theosophical Publishing House, 1976.

Vivekananda, Swami. *Karma Yoga: The Yoga of Action* (English translation). California: Vedanta Press, 1999.

Weiler, Linda Christy. Academy of Holistic Fitness Specialty Certificate Manual, 2009.

Williamson, Marianne. *A Course in Weight Loss: 21 Spiritual Lessons for Surrendering Your Weight Forever*. California: Hay House, 2010.

Index

Page numbers of illustrations appear in italics.

ABOUT THE AUTHOR

BETH SHAW is the founder and president of YogaFit Training Systems, the largest yoga school in North America. The leader in mind-body education, YogaFit has trained more than 250,000 fitness instructors on six continents. The author of *Beth Shaw's YogaFit*, Shaw has also created more than a dozen bestselling yoga and fitness DVDs. She writes a weekly column for *Parade*, and she and her company have been featured on television and in print, including CNBC, CNN, E!, and in *The New York Times, The Wall Street Journal, O: The Oprah Magazine, Time, More, Entrepreneur, Yoga Journal, Glamour, Self, USA Today, The Huffington Post*, and numerous fitness magazines. Although she gained her fame—and experience as an entrepreneur—from building YogaFit, Shaw is also an accomplished life coach, anger management specialist, and meditation teacher. Shaw holds a certification in business management from Long Island University and numerous mind-body modalities. She sits on the board of many nonprofit animal rights organizations and is an outspoken animal advocate. An international presenter and popular speaker, Shaw has lectured and taught on six continents. When not traveling, she splits her time between the Los Angeles area and New York City.

www.Bethshaw.com

Facebook.com/YogaFitTrainingSystemsWorldwide

@bethshawyoga